Run Healthy

The Runner's Guide to Injury Prevention and Treatment

Emmi Aguillard

Jonathan Cane

Allison Goldstein

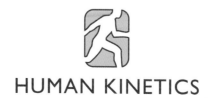

HUMAN KINETICS

Library of Congress Cataloging-in-Publication Data

Names: Aguillard, Emmi, 1991- author. | Cane, Jonathan, author. |
  Goldstein, Allison, 1986- author.
Title: Run healthy : the runner's guide to injury prevention and treatment
  / Emmi Aguillard, Jonathan Cane, Allison Goldstein.
Description: Champaign, IL : Human Kinetics, [2024] | Includes
  bibliographical references and index.
Identifiers: LCCN 2022041754 (print) | LCCN 2022041755 (ebook) | ISBN
  9781718203747 (paperback) | ISBN 9781718203754 (epub) | ISBN
  9781718203761 (pdf)
Subjects: LCSH: Running injuries--Prevention. | Running
  injuries--Treatment. | Running--Physiological aspects. | BISAC: SPORTS &
  RECREATION / Running & Jogging | HEALTH & FITNESS / Pain Management
Classification: LCC RC1220.R8 A38 2024 (print) | LCC RC1220.R8 (ebook) |
  DDC 617.1/0276425--dc23/eng/20220929
LC record available at https://lccn.loc.gov/2022041754
LC ebook record available at https://lccn.loc.gov/2022041755

ISBN: 978-1-7182-0374-7 (print)

Senior Acquisitions Editor: Michelle Earle; **Senior Developmental Editor:** Cynthia McEntire; **Managing Editor:** Kevin Matz; **Copyeditor:** E before I Editing; **Indexer:** Ferreira Indexing; **Permissions Manager:** Laurel Mitchell; **Senior Graphic Designer:** Sean Roosevelt; **Cover Designer:** Keri Evans; **Cover Design Specialist:** Susan Rothermel Allen; **Photograph (cover):** ©Mark Ryan Pfeffer, All Rights Reserved; **Photographs (interior):** Danny Weiss; **Photo Asset Manager:** Laura Fitch; **Photo Production Specialist:** Amy M. Rose; **Photo Production Manager:** Jason Allen; **Senior Art Manager:** Kelly Hendren; **Illustrations:** © Human Kinetics; **Printer:** Versa Press

We thank Finish Line Physical Therapy in New Rochelle, New York, for assistance in providing the location for the photo shoot for this book.

Human Kinetics books are available at special discounts for bulk purchase. Special editions or book excerpts can also be created to specification. For details, contact the Special Sales Manager at Human Kinetics.

Printed in the United States of America   10   9   8   7   6   5   4   3   2   1

The paper in this book is certified under a sustainable forestry program.

Human Kinetics	*United States and International*	*Canada*
1607 N. Market Street	Website: **US.HumanKinetics.com**	Website: **Canada.HumanKinetics.com**
Champaign, IL 61820	Email: info@hkusa.com	Email: info@hkcanada.com
USA	Phone: 1-800-747-4457	

E8314

To the coaches I had at a young age who instilled in me a lifelong love for this sport; my family (especially my mother, who helped this physical therapist become a writer); the mentors who have taught me both the importance of lifelong learning and how to care for, inspire, and be inspired by my patients; and every patient I've treated, from whom I've learned so much.

– Emmi

To my parents who believed in me, even when I didn't; to my wife and son, who inspire me and challenge me every day; to my athletes, who put their trust in me and allow me to do what I love.

– Jonathan

To every coach, scientist, and healthcare professional who lent me their expertise on my running and writing journeys.

– Allison

Contents

Acknowledgements

This book would not have been possible without the help, input, support, and professional expertise of even more people than we are able to name here.

We want to thank Alison McGinnis, Morgan Mowers, Cuyler Hudson, Rachelle Bordlee, and Darlene Aguillard for reading early drafts of many chapters of this book. You helped ensure that we brought the most current, useful exercises to athletes in a way that makes sense to them.

Likewise, we thank the Gray Institute and the Postural Restoration Institute for their contributions to the field of physical therapy and to our understanding of movement and rehabilitation. Thanks also to Lauren Antonucci of Nutrition Energy, for your valuable contributions to the nutrition content we have shared.

Thank you to Devang Patel, Chelsea Frengs, Ryan Pinerio, Nicole Sin Quee for dedicating your time and bodies to pose for the pages of this book, and Danny Weiss for brilliantly capturing the not-always-easy-to-explain poses that we requested. Thanks to Michael Conlon and Finish Line Physical Therapy for generously letting us use your state-of-the-art New Rochelle facility for our photo shoot, and thanks also to Rabbit and Brooks for outfitting our models.

Finally, we owe a great deal of thanks to Michelle Earle, Cynthia McEntire, and the entire publishing team at Human Kinetics. Without your tireless work (and patience), this book would not exist. We are thrilled to have worked with you to get such an important guide out of our heads and into the hands of runners who need it.

Introduction

Running is the world's oldest organized sport—and for good reason. Nothing could be simpler than putting one foot in front of the other. The Sports & Fitness Industry Association estimates there are more than 47 million runners in the United States, and it's the most popular participatory sport for middle school and high school athletes as well as adults. Young or old, big or small, fast or slow, people run for competition, for the numerous health benefits, and—believe it or not—for fun.

Yet as straightforward as running is, it's not without some inherent risks and challenges. If you've ever found yourself in pain while running, or if you've missed workouts because of injuries, you're far from alone. In fact, of those nearly 50 million American runners, about half of them were sidelined by an injury last year alone.

Although some injuries fall into the "nature of the beast" category, many can be avoided or minimized with a smart approach. If you get injured, quick diagnosis and prudent treatment can make the difference between an ailment that keeps you off the roads for a few days and one that's a season-ender. Everyone from weekend warriors to elite runners can benefit from a program that helps them address the cause of injuries as well as assists in their treatment.

In the pages that follow you'll find both clinical and practical information presented by a doctor of physical therapy who specializes in treating runners and endurance athletes and has been a runner herself for more than 20 years, competing in distances ranging from the 1500m at the D1 level to the Boston Marathon, and an exercise physiologist and coach who has worked with endurance athletes (including world champions and world record holders) for more than 30 years. Written for runners, as well as coaches, parents, and health professionals, *Run Healthy: The Runner's Guide to Injury Prevention and Treatment* helps the reader gain a better understanding of how the musculoskeletal system functions and responds to training, how to identify an injury, when rest is necessary (versus training through the injury), and when to seek professional treatment.

We start off with an anatomy overview, explaining the different types of tissue that make up the body's musculoskeletal system. From there, we take a deeper dive into some of the most common and frustrating injuries runners encounter. We show you how to identify, avoid, and treat everything from muscle strains to tendinitis, from stress fractures to iliotibial band syndrome. In addition to the clinical side of things, we take a look at common form issues that can lead to injury and how a combination of strength work, mobility exercises, and running drills can help you clean up your form and improve your running economy and performance. Finally, we offer some insight into alternative and complementary treatments, helping you separate fact from fiction.

Run Healthy: The Runner's Guide to Injury Prevention and Treatment includes anatomical drawings to help you understand the physiology, as well as photographs demonstrating the exercises and drills. We're confident that the combination of objective, clinical advice, coupled with practical anecdotes from our experience treating and coaching runners, will prepare you for years of healthy and productive miles.

Happy running!

Exercise Finder

Exercise	Page number	Warm-up	Cool-down	Mobility	Strength	Prehab	Rehab
Feet and toes							
Splay your feet	37			X	X	X	X
Toe yoga	38		X	X	X	X	X
Active assisted range of motion for toes	39			X	X	X	X
Arch stretch	40	X	X			X	X
Pronation driver	40	X	X			X	X
Arch activation: Supination driver and short foot	41	X					
Three-way balance driver	42	X					
Toe separators	44					X	
Ankles							
Soft tissue mobilization	53	X	X	X		X	X
Ankle massage	53	X		X		X	
3D calf stretch	54	X	X	X	X	X	X
3D banded strength exercises	55				X	X	X
Knees							
3D kneeling hip flexor stretch	64	X	X	X		X	X
Long arc quad	65				X	X	X
Single-leg split squat (Bulgarian split squat)	66	X			X	X	X
Lateral toe taps	67	X			X	X	X
Monster walks	67	X			X	X	X
Wall sit	71	X			X	X	X
Eccentric squat on an incline board	72				X		X
Double-leg squat	72				X	X	X
Single-leg squat	73				X	X	X
Box jumps	74				X	X	X
Multidirectional hops	74				X	X	X
Hips							
Foam rolling the glutes, TFL, and quads	86	X	X	X		X	X
Trigger point release: Hip flexor (psoas)	88	X	X	X		X	X
Hip floss	88			X		X	X
3D pivots	90	X		X		X	X
Common lunge matrix	92	X	X			X	X

(continued)

PART I
THE RUNNER'S BODY

CHAPTER 1

Understanding the Body's Tissues and Their Healing Processes

Before we delve into the specific injuries that affect runners, let's get a sense of what our bodies are made of. Understanding the different types of tissues that make up our musculoskeletal system, in particular, is critical to understanding what is malfunctioning and, in turn, how the body will heal. In this chapter, we'll differentiate muscle, tendons and ligaments, bones, and connective tissue. As you read about specific injuries later in the book—for instance, a muscle strain versus a bone stress injury—you can better identify them and recognize what can be done to heal injuries and prevent them from occurring again.

Geography of the Body

When we think about the human body and its different internal structures, it can be helpful to think of it as a topographical map. Although the earth's mountains, oceans, plains, and deserts are interconnected and unmarked, topographers have labeled them so that we can navigate and understand the world we live in. Scientists, likewise, have mapped out the human body. And just as sometimes there are no physical boundaries that correspond with a country's made-up borders, the human body also exists as a continuum: Muscles morph into tendons, which connect to bones. These structures have a lot in common, but they also have distinct differences. We will explore both similarities and differences in this chapter.

Muscle

Muscles are the power generators of our body. They are what enable every movement we make, from an individual heartbeat to the thousands of steps it takes to run a marathon. Let's look at the basic composition and function of muscles as we journey down the road of injury, resilience, and performance.

Muscle Composition

Muscles are made up of countless individual fibers (figure 1.1), which are the contractile units that your brain can tell to shorten in order to generate force and power. Muscles are highly vascularized, meaning that they have an incredibly rich blood supply. This allows oxygen and nutrients to be delivered very quickly to muscle tissue, which aids exercise recovery and injury rehabilitation because blood delivers what tissues—including muscles—need to heal.

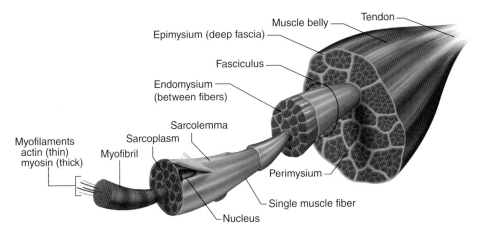

Figure 1.1   Structure of skeletal muscle.

Muscle Contraction

Muscles contract in three basic ways (figure 1.2). All are critical for performance and are integral in strength training. If you are recovering from a muscular injury, the muscle tissue will be able to tolerate different types of contractions at different points in the healing process.

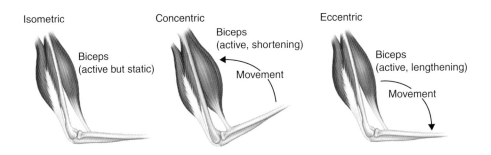

Figure 1.2   Types of muscle contraction.

An *isometric* muscle contraction occurs when a muscle contracts without any actual movement of the body. Think of squeezing a ball in your fist or pushing against a wall: No movement occurs, but a force is present. These types of muscle contractions enhance blood flow to muscles and can be incorporated early on in the rehab process to promote tissue healing (Neumann 2010).

A *concentric* muscle contraction occurs when the muscle fibers shorten or move closer together. A simple example of this is a calf raise. An example from running is the contraction of the calf muscle as you push off the ground, propelling your body forward. When recovering from an injury, concentric is usually the second type of contraction that the tissue can handle safely.

An *eccentric* muscle contraction occurs when a muscle contracts as it is being stretched or lengthened. This often occurs when you're trying to resist gravity. Think of slowly lowering your arm to put a glass down, controlling a squat with your quadriceps muscles as you sink lower, or absorbing the shock of impact with your quad muscles (as your knee bends) when running. Eccentric contractions are the strongest type of contraction, but because the forces involved are generally greater than in other types of contractions, they can be damaging for healing tissue (Neumann 2010). The benefits of eccentric muscle contraction can't be overstated when realigning tissue fibers, promoting blood flow to injured tissue, increasing resiliency, and reducing the risk of reinjury to specific body parts. However, eccentric contractions can be counterproductive to the recovery process if done too soon.

Triplanar Movement

The role of muscle contraction is to move our bones and joints in any of three planes of motion (figure 1.3). Not every joint will move in all three planes; some of our joints are designed for stability (knee), while others are designed for mobility (hip, ankle). Yet to thoroughly understand movement and running, we need to attend to all three planes of motion.

The first is the sagittal plane—flexion and extension (think "front to back"). This is the primary plane of motion in which we run. The second is the frontal plane, which is adduction and abduction, or side to side. Finally, the transverse (or horizontal) plane is where we get

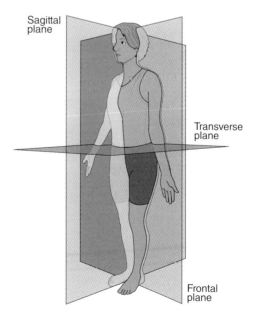

Figure 1.3 Three planes of motion: sagittal, frontal, and transverse.

rotation, both internal and external. While running is primarily a sagittal plane movement, there are significant components of both frontal and transverse plane movement, and weaknesses or restrictions in these planes can drive injury, which we will address throughout this book.

Specific to running, the hip and the ankle joint are designed to move in all three planes of motion, so they need adequate mobility for the joints to move from front to back, from side to side, and rotationally. The knee joint, on the other hand, is primarily intended to function in the sagittal plane. However, lack of mobility in the regions above and below the knee can cause compensation and excessive torque at the knee joint; this is a prime driver for injury. As you're working through the book and come across various triplanar exercises, now you'll know why!

Injury to Muscle Tissue

When we train, we develop small microtears in our muscles—this is part of why we experience soreness after a tough workout. As the body works to repair the damaged tissue, those muscle cells grow back bigger and stronger than they were before, so they're more resilient the next time you stress them that way. This explains why optimizing recovery is so important: You don't actually become stronger *during* training, but in the time *between* efforts when your body is repairing itself and increasing tissue resilience. For now, all you need to know is that if there are continued microtears to the muscle without adequate recovery time, injury is more likely to occur.

Tendons and Ligaments

Tendons and ligaments connect muscle to bone and bone to bone, respectively. Tendons and ligaments are made of connective tissue (figure 1.4), which can be thought of as a rope: It's a whole lot stronger than a muscle, and its job is to attach other tissues to one another, specifically bone.

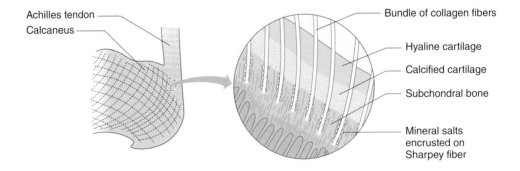

Figure 1.4 Tendon to bone connection, specifically the connection of the Achilles tendon to the calcaneus (anklebone).

In true rope fashion, connective tissue is made up of dense, parallel collagen fibers, leaving (compared to muscles) little room for blood vessels (figure 1.5). This parallel orientation gives tendons the ability to transfer large loads or forces between an active muscle and the joint into which it inserts—forces greater than a muscle or the joint alone could handle without injury. The same orientation enables ligaments to resist forces that try to stretch it in multiple directions. Tendons and ligaments that often cause runners trouble are the Achilles tendon, the patellar tendon, and the ligaments in the ankle, which are associated with ankle sprain.

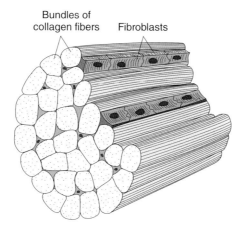

Figure 1.5   Parallel orientation of collagen fibers.

Tendons

Although similar in structure and composition, tendons and ligaments differ in their function. Tendons help with efficient load transfer—a property referred to as *elastic recoil* or *viscoelasticity* of the tissue. Imagine a rubber band. When the rubber band is pulled back, it starts to store elastic energy, or passive tension. *Passive* is key—this is how we produce power without expending additional energy. Tension progressively increases until the muscle and tendon reach a very high level of stiffness. There is an optimal length–tension relationship, and it is here that we want to release the muscle (rubber band) to use it for increased power and function. We see this in running when we land, hit the ground, and immediately bound forward: We are using elastic recoil for propulsion.

When a tendon is subject to a large force, it needs to be able to lengthen to effectively transfer energy. For example, the Achilles tendon can elongate up to 10 percent of its resting length with maximum calf contraction. This allows the body to store and release energy during running and jumping, and it protects against forces that could cause injury. If the force is too large, the tendon can't lengthen the way it needs to. That's when we run into problems. Following smart training principles and incorporating resistance training are essential to strengthen the tendon and increase its load capacity to help it better adapt to the demands of training and reduce risk of injury. We will cover how to accomplish both throughout this book.

Ligaments

Rather than helping with efficient energy or load transfer, ligaments are protective in nature. We rely on them for stabilization. When excessive force is applied to a joint and movement at that joint needs to be limited—for example, to avoid an ankle sprain or knee twist—that's when ligaments get to work. Ligaments are central to our body's ability to stabilize and resist against various external forces, and they function optimally when a stretch is applied to them. After the initial slack is pulled tight, the tissue provides immediate tension that restrains motion at a joint or between two bones.

If there is ligamentous laxity—loose ligaments caused by injury, disease, or trauma (such as repeated ankle sprains or the stress of pregnancy and childbirth)—muscles take over and play a more dominant role in providing our body with stability. Muscles around the joint that has gone lax will tighten to provide stability. However, muscles are not as quick to respond to external forces as ligaments, and that lag can lead to further injury. Accurately identifying the underlying issue leads to properly rehabilitating the structures. If you keep treating a chronic muscle injury, but the problem is actually a lax ligament, you'll just keep getting reinjured.

Injury and Repair

The composition of tendons and ligaments is what makes injury to them so frustrating. As mentioned earlier, adequate blood flow is how the body heals and repairs damaged tissues, so a part of the body that has less vascularization (blood flow) will take longer to heal. Because tendons and ligaments have a lesser supply of blood vessels and vascularization than muscles do, healing and rehabilitating tendon or ligament injuries takes longer.

When injury or damage to a tendon or ligament occurs, the parallel collagen fibers tear, and scar tissue forms. As the body repairs these fibers, due to the scar tissue, they are no longer aligned in the strong, resilient, parallel form they once were. Consequently, appropriate rehabilitation requires specific exercises to promote blood flow and realign the fibers to rebuild resilience and prevent reinjury.

Knowing the correct way to rehabilitate a tendon or ligament injury is critical. You may have been frustrated when, after taking two weeks off from running due to Achilles pain, your pain came right back. Or maybe you have experienced tendinitis that seemed to feel better after you ran. The reason these things can happen is that, somewhat counterintuitively (especially if you've had muscle or bone injuries in the past that required complete rest), incorporating exercises, modalities, and strategies that increase blood flow to the damaged region is the most effective way to help the body heal. An immobilized tendon or ligament will not receive adequate blood flow to heal; therefore, rest alone is rarely the answer for this type of injury. In order to facilitate healing in a tendon or ligament, exercises that promote increased blood flow to the region while loading the tissue submaximally (i.e., with less force than what caused the injury but with enough force to help the tissue to heal) is critical. This is also why these injuries can be so tough to overcome; the injured tendon or ligament requires enough stress to stimulate healing, but too much can cause an increase in inflammation, which is counterproductive. This line is very fine. We are going to get more specific in upcoming chapters about how to do this for a few of the most common running injuries, but these same principles apply to the entire body.

Bone

Bone is a superspecialized connective tissue, made up of calcium, collagen, and salts that form a hard, dense structure that serves as the rigid support framework for our body. Yet despite its rigid composition, bone is extremely dynamic. Of all the different tissues in our body, bone has the best capacity for remodeling, repair, and regeneration. This is in large part due to a uniquely rich blood supply, which allows the tissue to constantly adapt in response to physical stress.

Bone lays down more bone in areas of high stress and reabsorbs bone in areas of low stress. Commonly known as Wolff's law, this concept helps us understand how the body heals. Each time you run, the pounding of your feet against pavement creates tiny microfractures in your bones. Wolff's law tells us that when this occurs, the body lays down more bone to build resilience to this physical stress, adapting to this increased load and force. Where we can get into trouble is when we don't allow enough time for this healing process to occur between bouts of physical stress (e.g., runs). A common occurrence is runners ramping up their mileage too quickly and developing stress fractures. It takes *years* for the body to adapt to the demands of running; it's not a process that can be rushed. And because bone is the densest tissue in our bodies, it is also the slowest to adapt to training and the slowest to heal from injury.

Connective Tissue: Fasciae and Bursae

Connective tissue has historically been neglected when it comes to the study of anatomy, but in recent years, more research is pointing to the critical role that connective tissue plays in athletic performance. The primary connective tissue in the body is fascia, which is composed mostly of collagen and elastin—two proteins that serve as the building blocks for much of our mus-culoskeletal system. Fascia *surrounds* each muscle, exists *within* the different muscle fibers of each muscle, and is also continuous *across* muscles, meaning that contracting one muscle will pull on the connective fascia and affect the tension of another muscle. Fascia is responsible for the structure of each muscle, serves as a conduit for blood vessels and nerves, and provides the critical passive tension needed for the elastic recoil mechanism we described earlier—in a nutshell, fascia provides structural support and elasticity to our muscles. When a muscle contracts, connective tissue is what transfers this force to the tendon and joint, enabling our overall movement. Without connective tissue, we wouldn't be moving at all!

A specialized type of connective tissue is a bursa, a term worth mention-ing because many doctors love throwing around the term *bursitis* to label inflammation that occurs in various parts of the body, most commonly the knee or hip. What is a bursa? It's a fluid-filled sac whose role is to reduce friction by enabling one structure to move freely over another. Bursae exist throughout our body to help facilitate smooth movement between skin and bony prominences such as the elbow or knee, beneath deep fascia, and between tendons and bones. Restrictions in this specific type of connective tissue can lead to inflammation of the bursae, causing pain in the structure or undue stress on the tendon or bone that it is intended to help support (Moore, Daly, and Agur 2010).

Conclusion

Tissues don't exist in isolation. In our basic biology classes, we are taught that tendon connects muscle to bone. In reality, it's more like muscle gradu-ally turns into tendon, tendons join with and attach to bone, and a chain of connective tissue impacts all of these components simultaneously. Because of this intricate connectivity, a thorough understanding of the body's anatomi-cal framework is our starting point for rehabilitation and injury prevention.

Injury occurs when too much force is applied to a structure of the body and that structure fails. As we delve into the biomechanics of running and form in chapter 16, you'll come to understand each component of your form. If one structure of your body is consistently undergoing more force or strain than another due to restrictions in movement or biomechanical errors, injury is more likely to occur. That's why giving equal attention to mobility work, strength training, biomechanics, and form is critical for a runner.

CHAPTER 2

Navigating Your Treatment Options

Now that you have a basic understanding of the components of the musculoskeletal system, let's break down the intended use of this book. First and foremost, this book is not intended to replace evaluation and treatment from a medical professional. Rather, the goal is to help you better understand your body and the causes of common injuries and learn to avoid common running mistakes. We will take you through each region of the body, limb by limb, with loads of tips and tricks on prevention and self-management of injuries. That way, you can spend less time dealing with injuries and more time dedicated to enjoying your favorite pastime.

The value of prevention, or prehab, is priceless, and nipping a small annoyance in the bud before it turns into a full-blown injury is our ultimate goal. An inch of prevention really does go a mile (or a marathon!), and addressing some areas that might be a bit overworked—or underworked—can save you a lot of grief. It may even prevent you from having to miss your morning run.

What exactly is prehab? Here's a simple example. Say your calves are always really tight after you finish a run. Left untreated, this might eventually lead to Achilles tendinitis. But, by acknowledging that your calves are working too hard, giving them a little bit of tender loving care (TLC) with foam rolling or soft tissue maintenance, and helping them to recover better, you will save yourself a lot of grief.

But wait, this isn't enough! TLC to the calves alone won't fix you. We need to step back and look at the bigger picture to figure out *why* those calves are working too hard. Are your hip flexors too tight, preventing hip extension and causing you to push off mainly from your calf? Are your glutes weak, preventing you from getting enough drive from higher up in the posterior chain? We will break down all of this for you in the pages of this book. Injuries need to be treated twofold: First look locally at the body part that's bothered, and then look globally for why it's bothered. Ultimately, prehab is addressing that "why" before it can cause pain and injury to the body part that would eventually bear the brunt of the dysfunction. It's a relatively small investment in your health that can help prevent or minimize running-related injuries.

Common running injuries can be separated into two basic categories. An area becomes injured either because it's overworked and overly fatigued or because it's underworked and weak. Sometimes, the injury can be a combination of the two; perhaps a certain area that is being overworked is also weak. That means double trouble. Later chapters in this book will help you determine which category your injury fits into and ways to manage the fatigue or weakness. (And yes, there's a third category: accident! We cover some of these less common, acute injuries, too.)

When to Get Help

As a runner, you are probably asking yourself, "Is this pain or injury something that I can run through or do I need to shut things down? Is this something that I can handle myself, or is it time to see a professional?"

A good place to start is to identify where you are on the pain scale. This can help you to screen yourself and determine if an injury is appropriate to run through or if it is severe enough to need some rest. The golden rule of when you can run is that if your pain is less than a 3 out of 10 (on a scale with 0 being no pain and 10 being "please take me to the hospital"), you have the green light to head out for your run (figure 2.1). But this is not the only guide. If your pain increases as you run or if you feel yourself compensating (changing your stride), *stop*. This is not something you want to run through. Grab your handy running injury bible, swap today's run for a cross-training day (probably tomorrow, too), and let's get busy figuring out this injury and nipping it in the bud.

Although it might seem counterintuitive, rest alone is rarely the answer when it comes to running injuries. Tissues require movement, healthy stress, and modulated exercise to receive the blood flow and circulation required to promote full healing and to regain the strength needed in the affected region to return to running. That said, it *is* appropriate to rest an injury when it is severe enough to require attention from a medical professional. If you are unable to walk without compensating or are waking up during the night due to pain or discomfort, it's time to seek outside treatment. Other red flags to look out for are a *lack* of feeling in an area (numbness), significant and recent onset of weakness (like difficulty flexing your foot), or a distinct change in

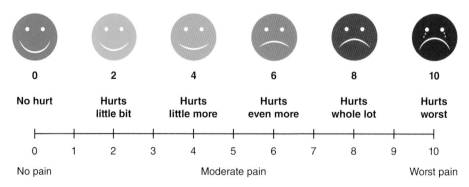

Figure 2.1   Pain scale.

coloring (the tissue has gone white or turned purple, blue, or black)—these could indicate a serious nerve or arterial issue, and you should seek medical treatment immediately.

Consulting an Expert

If you've determined that your injury or pain necessitates a medical professional, don't wait until the pain gets worse. However, it can be confusing to determine whom to contact. Even understanding what different types of medical professionals do can be overwhelming. Let's review the types of musculoskeletal health professionals you might work with and what they offer so that you can use this book as a reference to get you to the right expert if further treatment is needed. Assembling the appropriate team to address a serious or chronic injury can be a game changer.

Medical Doctor (MD, DO)

If you are having trouble walking or are experiencing pain that is present at rest, is waking you up during the night, or is impacting your life in any way outside of running, it's time to visit the doctor. You might be referred to an orthopedist or orthopedic surgeon. We highly recommend seeing a doctor who specializes in sports medicine; it's even better if they have experience working with runners or are runners themselves. When seeing a medical doctor, a sports orthopedist is a great choice. They will be able to order an MRI or X-ray to give you a better idea of what's going on in the injured area. They can also help you determine the best course of action, be it physical therapy, rest, or surgery for more serious injuries.

A word of caution: Your pain and what shows up in medical imaging are not always correlated. Just because an MRI indicates an abnormal result does not mean that this abnormality is the driver of your pain. Conversely, you can sometimes have pain without anything unusual showing up on the MRI. As an athlete, don't become overly focused on imaging; instead, treat your injury based on your level of function. How much is the pain affecting your running? How is your joint mobility and muscle strength? An example of this is a labral injury. Often, an MRI of the hip will reveal a labral tear as a secondary finding in a patient being treated for another issue, such as hamstring tendinitis or iliotibial band syndrome. The labral tear is not contributing to the patient's pain, and it's likely that imaging of the uninjured hip would show the same thing. (It's estimated that 40 to 60 percent of us have a labral injury; in fact, in Europe they don't even report labral injury on MRI findings because it's not considered significant.) Yet, a labral injury *can* cause pain if it's inflamed, and doctors will even do surgery on the hip labrum in certain cases. Two runners could present with the exact same imaging, but one is symptomatic and the other isn't. This leads us to a deeper dive into the runner's hip mechanics, which we will address in chapter 8.

Physical Therapist (PT)

You can usually save yourself a step in the medical appointment process if you head straight to a physical therapist. All 50 states now allow you direct access to a physical therapist, meaning you can see a PT without a doctor's referral or prescription. Your physical therapist will be able to evaluate your injury; rule out more serious issues; assess your strength, gait, and movement patterns; get you started with tailored strategies to alleviate pain and symptoms; and prescribe strength exercises to address the underlying dysfunction. PTs have been trained in differential diagnosis, which means they are able to determine when following up with an MD for imaging, medication, surgery, or injections might be necessary. We recommend starting with a PT as a more direct, streamlined approach to injury, followed by a visit to the MD if you don't make progress in returning to your normal activities.

Other Professionals: Chiropractor, Acupuncturist, Massage Therapist

Chiropractors, acupuncturists, and massage therapists are trained professionals who each use different methodologies to treat acute pain and inflammation, break up soft tissue and joint restrictions, and help you get to a state where you are able to function pain-free. For many athletes, they are a key step in the rehabilitation process. Sometimes it's impossible to make the necessary form or strength changes if your pain is preventing you from moving or if your body is so stiff that you can't access the regions that need to move.

When choosing any of these alternative treatment options, we recommend looking for a provider who specializes in working with sports injuries and athletes, specifically runners.

Chiropractor

Chiropractors use treatments that overlap with physical therapists including modalities such as EPAT (extracorporeal pulse activation technology, which uses acoustic pressure waves), laser therapy, and other technologies that help increase blood flow and circulation to a particular region. These can be good options for dealing with a pesky injury, especially as an intervention before getting surgery. If you experience severe joint restrictions that limit proper movement, high-velocity joint manipulations—in which chiropractors specialize—can be the key to unlocking certain regions of your body (thoracic spine or ankle mobility, for example). You may then have a better canvas for your strength and form work to succeed in improving your movement patterns.

Acupuncturist

While there is no consensus about the efficacy of acupuncture among health professionals, acupuncturists may be useful providers to help with pain management, especially if you have chronic pain or if several different systems are involved with your injury. Acupuncture involves the use of very thin needles placed into your skin at specific locations. The procedure can help to release soft tissue restrictions, reduce inflammation, and improve circulation to chronically injured areas. It may also downregulate the nervous system, increase your body's parasympathetic activity, and improve overall tension. In chapter 18 we do a deeper dive into the pros and cons of acupuncture.

Massage Therapist

Massage therapy is another treatment option, especially if you are needle averse. Deep tissue work can help improve blood flow and circulation, decrease lactic acid accumulation, improve joint mobility, reduce edema and swelling, increase fascial mobility and glide, and reduce pain. Working with a therapist who specializes in deep tissue sports massage therapy will likely give the best results.

Registered Dietitian (RD)

Chapter 17 is fully devoted to nutrition, but we want to touch on the value of working with a dietitian here as well. Exercise, strength, proper training, and biomechanics are only half the battle of training; it is impossible for your body to heal if you aren't fueling properly. Adding a registered dietitian to your medical provider team can be valuable. As you look for a provider, be aware that registered dietitians (RDs) have a master's degree, partake in an extended internship, and sit for board exams—they complete extensive training to earn their credentials. On the other hand, people who label themselves as nutritionists are not held to such strict standards; almost anyone can complete a nutrition certificate program and call themselves a nutritionist. When seeking nutrition advice, be sure to search for an RD to assist with your needs.

Conclusion

Runners may respond differently than their peers to different types of treatment, and there is often overlap between providers. Your running buddy may swear by their acupuncturist, whereas you might find the most benefit from a massage therapist. It can take some experimentation to find the best option for your body and your injury. Often, a combination of treatments can be the best solution. Be patient as you explore what works for you.

Now we're ready to dive into what might cause you pain or injury when running. We will take you through your body region by region, starting at the feet and working all the way up through the spine. In each chapter, you'll find a breakdown of the anatomy of each region, common running injuries (with case examples), and treatment approaches specific to each body part. Use this information to help you decide how best to manage those aches and pains that come up suddenly or never seem to completely go away. We want to help you learn to run pain-free for the long haul.

CHAPTER 3

Injuries to Muscle and Bone

As discussed in chapter 1, muscles, tendons, and bones have unique properties that differentiate and dictate the time frame of healing. Rest alone does not always result in complete healing. Here we outline the principles of healing for each of these tissue types.

Muscle and Tendon Injuries

One of the biggest nightmares for a runner is the dreaded "pop" while on a run. A muscle injury might also present as a sudden, sharp pain that changes our stride, sometimes forcing us to limp home. This sensation usually indicates some degree of tearing within a muscle or tendon. Several words are used to describe this type of injury—strain, sprain, tear, pull—but the medical community uses "tear" across the board and applies a graded system to classify its severity (figure 3.1).

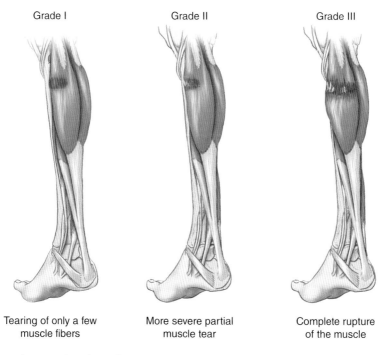

Grade I — Tearing of only a few muscle fibers

Grade II — More severe partial muscle tear

Grade III — Complete rupture of the muscle

Figure 3.1 Three grades of muscles tears.

A grade-1 tear (pull or strain) is categorized as mild damage to individual muscle fibers in which fewer than 5 percent of muscle fibers are torn. Usually a runner will experience soreness and some decreased strength, but little bruising or loss of function. Grade-1 tears usually take two to four weeks to heal. A runner is often able to continue training at reduced volume and intensity, but we recommend consulting with a physical therapist or MD prior to resuming activity. Incorporating speed work or hill training too soon can very easily result in reinjury of the muscle very easily.

A grade 2 tear involves roughly 5 to 50 percent of the muscle or tendon being torn or damaged and results in greater loss of strength and function. These injuries can take two to three months to heal, and recovery requires more rest and activity modification. A runner will have pain with muscle contraction and present with decreased strength and range of motion. Running through this injury is *not* advised, although you may be able to continue with cross-training such as swimming or biking, depending on the specifics of your injury.

A grade 3 tear involves greater than 50 percent of the muscle or tendon, resulting in almost complete loss of function. Gapping may occur—a gap appears as a dent under the skin where ripped pieces of muscle start to separate—and a runner will have little or no ability to contract the injured muscle. In severe cases of grade 3 tears, surgery is required.

Tears may happen in the muscle belly but more commonly occur at the muscle–tendon junction, where the blood-filled contractile muscle fibers meet the strong, ropy collagen tendon. A tear that occurs within the tendon or at muscle–tendon junction is slower to heal than a tear that occurs within the muscle belly because of the reduced blood supply to the tendon. Advanced rehab will most likely be required for a tendon injury to regain full function.

Runners and athletes are more likely to injure a muscle if they are limited in strength and flexibility or if they are exerting themselves while fatigued (e.g., at the end of a tough workout or race). Injury is also more likely to occur in a muscle that crosses two joints, such as the hamstrings, quadriceps, and calf muscles, all major players in the running gait cycle. Diligence with strength and mobility while training reduces injury in these areas.

Treatment of Muscle and Tendon Injury

Muscle and tendon injuries are some of the trickiest to rehab on your own. Do too much, and you'll aggravate the injury, increase inflammation, and potentially make things worse, which delays healing. Do too little, on the other hand, and the healing trajectory is going to plateau—remember, tissues respond to stress! It's a fine line between the two, and there are many different factors that can change where this line is, even on a day-to-day basis. (How much did you do the day before? Did you get a good night of sleep? Are you well hydrated?) Our job is to help you navigate that line, but there may come a time when professional help is needed. Here is a generalized timeline for treatment.

Acute Phase: Week One

Traditional treatment of acute muscle injury is commonly referred to as RICE (rest, ice, compress, and elevate) and also includes nonsteroidal anti-inflammatory drugs (NSAIDs). Many doctors are quick to prescribe these as the first line of defense to a new or acute muscle injury. After one or two weeks of rest, physical therapy should be assigned in order to regain full function.

Though RICE is a long-standing standard of care, recent evidence suggests a shift in acute management of muscle injury. There is little evidence to support the use of ice in acute injury for anything more than pain relief. Ice may still be recommended within the first few hours following injury to reduce inflammation, but only for short periods of time. A suggestion is icing for 15 minutes with at least 30 minutes between each session for the first 24 to 48 hours following injury.

Anti-inflammatories are similarly controversial. Acute inflammation is your body's natural healing response, and there are differing opinions on if taking NSAIDS in the acute phase of injury is indeed the best protocol.

Heat can be a useful tool in the acute phase of muscle injury specifically. The body will often react to a strain by tensing the surrounding muscle. Heat can help reduce this tension, which can take pressure off the injured area. Heat also promotes increased blood flow to the area.

Although taking time off from running helps you heal and avoid compensating in ways that create other mechanical issues, total rest can lead to increased stiffness and atrophy. Even in the acute phase of muscle injury, isometrics (contraction without movement, just resistance) along with gentle range-of-motion exercises are recommended if these exercises do not cause further pain. Do not be afraid to use "motion as lotion"—gentle, pain-free movements can help speed recovery by increasing blood flow to injured areas. Keeping an area pliable and protecting range of motion will give your body a jump start on the healing process and prevent scar tissue from forming. As always, it is never a good idea to push through pain unless under the supervision of a medical professional.

Subacute Phase: Two to Four Weeks Post-Injury

After the first two or three weeks of rehabilitation, focus shifts to safely regaining strength. When a muscle tears, the body inhibits us from using the injured area too much, and weakness and atrophy are quick to follow. First things first: Regain full range of motion. Then progress to strengthening and load tolerance via isometric, concentric, and eccentric strengthening. Finally, reintroduce plyometric training.

Concentric muscle contraction is the shortening of a muscle (think of a biceps curl). Calf raises for a calf strain, hamstring curls and bridges for hamstring injury, or straight-leg raises for the quad are examples of concen-

Cortisone: Yes or No?

Although physicians sometimes offer cortisone shots as quick fixes for muscle injuries, we recommend that they should be used only as a last resort. Inflammation is the body's healing response to an injury; both NSAIDs and cortisone, to varying degrees, can halt the body's healing processes. While they do provide temporary relief from pain and a temporary increase in function, they may weaken the integrity of a tendon in the long run by preventing the appropriate healing mechanisms from reaching the injury. When the healing process is disrupted in this manner, the body may never fully heal the injured region.

A safer and more restorative course of action is to use regenerative modalities to promote and enhance the body's own natural healing processes. Examples of these modalities are heat for at-home application and laser therapy or platelet-rich plasma injections for clinical application.

tric exercises. These exercises can be progressively loaded with additional weight to tolerance.

Eccentric muscle contraction exercises should not be performed too early in the healing process, because they are the most load you can apply to a muscle—and often the type of contraction that caused your injury. But they are critical for building resilience and reducing your risk for reinjury. The slow, controlled lengthening of a muscle can help realign collagen fibers and prevent scar tissue from forming.

Once a runner can perform eccentric muscle activities pain-free, plyometric training (hops and running drills) can be reintroduced. A return-to-running program should be discussed with your coach or physical therapist.

Prevention of Muscle Injury

Regular loading of the muscles and tendons through strength exercises is critical to preventing injury in the sport of running. This keeps the muscles and tendons happy, strong, and resilient enough to handle all the miles you might throw at them. We provide specific strength-building exercises throughout the book; a number of them can be found in chapters 7, 8, 9, and 13.

In addition to strength, maintaining adequate mobility is key. While a tight muscle is a strong muscle (the tighter a muscle, the more power it can produce), a tight muscle is also at increased risk of tearing. Rolling, stretching, and soft tissue maintenance can reduce your risk of tearing.

Bony Stress Injury

Stress fracture is a much-feared term to any runner because there is no shortcut or trick for training through one. Stress fractures respond best to rest. The goal, therefore, is to avoid them altogether. In this section, we highlight common risk factors for bony stress injury. This is not an injury to try to work through on your own. See your doctor as soon as possible if you suspect this is what you are dealing with.

Bone is the strongest structure in the body, so an injury here is slower to heal than most other running injuries. The silver lining of a bony stress injury is that although bone is slow to heal, with proper rest the likelihood of reinjuring a fully healed bony injury is slim. Bones heal well, and they heal relatively simply. Your body doesn't produce fibrous scar tissue within a bone; it simply builds more bone. For proper healing to occur, it is critical to reduce loading to the injured region and also to make sure you are getting adequate fuel to help the body reproduce the bone that it needs to lay down.

What exactly is a stress fracture? A stress fracture occurs if a bone is placed under too much load and the supporting muscles around it can no longer adequately absorb the load or impact. A stress fracture usually begins with swelling or inflammation inside of the bone, known as bony edema. If you were to get an MRI, a doctor might diagnose you with a stress reaction at this stage. Once there is fluid within a bone, the strength and integrity of the bone is compromised, and a runner is much more prone to a stress fracture, i.e., a small crack in the bone. Bones are intended to be strong and sturdy. Fluid within the bone creates a softness that can't withstand force to the same degree.

In runners, the most common place for stress fractures are in the metatarsal bones (foot) and in the tibia (shin). Stress fractures also occur in the femur and pelvis, although these are less common. While training error or form can be a major contributor to bony stress injury, stress fractures, especially those in larger bones such as the femur and pelvis, can be a telltale sign that a runner is underfueling.

Nutrition and Bony Injury

While calcium and vitamin D are famous for bone health, evidence supports an overall lack of caloric intake to be the driving factor for recurrent stress fractures, especially in female runners (Heikura et al. 2018). If a runner is not fueling enough postrun, the body will start to break down bone in order to meet its nutritional needs, and this paves the way to bone injury. Read chapter 17 to learn more about how nutrition can contribute to injury—and to healing.

A warning sign of a stress fracture can be a consistent dull ache that does not go away as you warm up and may get worse as you run. You may also notice increased tightness in the muscles surrounding the site of injury as your body tenses up to try to protect the region. Pain that is palpable at a small, isolated spot along the inside of your shin bone or on your foot could also be a sign that you have a bony injury.

The hop test can be a useful diagnostic tool. Jump and try to land heavily on your foot. If this provokes pain (more with landing than with pushing off), chances are high that you are dealing with bony injury.

The stakes are high here. If you continue to run on a stress fracture, you risk a full-blown fracture, i.e., a snap or break of the bone, which may require surgery. If it's a femoral neck or pelvic stress fracture, the risk of a complete break is significant. A fracture in your pelvis can result in an intensive surgery requiring metal hardware to be drilled into the hip to put the pieces of bone back together. A fracture to the femoral neck can tear the blood vessels that supply blood to the femoral head (the ball in the ball-and-socket of your hip bone), which can cause the bone tissue to die, a term coined *avascular necrosis*. Eventually, the entire bone can collapse. It's not advised to train through any of these.

Risk Factors in Female Runners

Women are more at risk than men for bony injury, especially runners who have experienced amenorrhea (loss of or an irregular menstrual cycle). Amenorrhea is a sign that your body is not getting enough nutrients, and there is a significant correlation between nutrient deficiencies and risk for stress fractures. Low estrogen levels can also inhibit your body from rebuilding bone. Low-estrogen birth control taken over a long time can decrease your body's overall estrogen levels enough to impact bone health. Working with your doctor and a registered dietitian is critical if you are amenorrheic or have low estrogen. The bottom line here is: If you aren't getting your period, this is a warning sign from your body. It is not a normal side effect of training. Period.

Prevention of Stress Fractures

How does one increase running volume while also reducing our risk of developing this pesky injury? There are several controllable factors you can implement as a part of your training to reduce the risk of developing a stress fracture.

First, gradually increase your volume to give your body and bones adequate time to adapt to the impact. Don't increase your mileage too quickly; give the bone time to adapt. Every time you run, it produces tiny microfractures in your bones. This is to be expected. Between runs, the body heals these microfractures, lays down more bone, and creates resilience. If the load is too great or there isn't enough recovery between efforts, stress fractures will occur.

Second, opt for softer training surfaces, such as a track or dirt trail, as often as possible. Running on a soft surface can be a game changer. It reduces the amount of force being absorbed by your body. This can help you safely increase your mileage while reducing impact on your bones.

Third, make sure that you are consuming enough calcium, vitamin D, and calories in general. If you are underfueling, your body will start to pull nutrients from your bones to use as fuel. If you've suffered from several stress fractures over the course of your running history, see a doctor for an evaluation. There may be an issue with your body's ability to absorb these vitamins and minerals. More than anything, however, evidence supports that getting enough caloric intake can make the biggest difference in reducing your risk of bony injury.

Finally, pay attention to form. Overstriding results in increased force throughout your entire lower body. Working to increase a slow cadence and land with your foot underneath your center of mass will reduce the amount of load going through your body with each step. (We recommend drills to make these corrections in chapter 16.) If you've had recurrent stress fractures in the same area and have addressed the issues we have discussed, there may be something going on mechanically with your form. It is worth seeing a physical therapist or coach who can evaluate your running form and help you work on your gait.

Conclusion

As with all injuries, muscle and bone injuries are best avoided. However, if you do experience one, it's essential that you properly diagnose it so you know whether you are safe to continue with light training (as with a grade-1 muscle tear) or whether full rest is necessary (as with a stress fracture). Prevention requires a gradual, rather than abrupt, accumulation of miles; strength training; and proper nutrition. Later chapters will address all these strategies, and more.

CHAPTER 4

Soft Tissue Maintenance

The running world is full of colorful buzzwords and phrases like *drop the hammer*, *hit the wall*, *bonk*, and our personal favorites, *LSD* (long slow distance) and *fartlek* workouts. These are some of the most fun and expressive ones, but they're not clinical terms, just jargon used by runners and coaches. On the other hand, the term *soft tissue* is used by medical professionals and is also thrown around by runners. Yet in some cases, it's probably misused or misunderstood by those runners. So before we talk about soft tissue maintenance, let's make sure we're all on the same page about what soft tissue is.

In casual conversation with runners, soft tissue usually refers to muscles, as well as fasciae, tendons, and ligaments. (If you're getting ready for medical school and your professor asks you to define soft tissue, be sure to include blood vessels, fat, nerves, and even your heart, but when your massage therapist talks about soft tissue work, it's a good bet they're not talking about massaging your ticker.) Soft tissue therapy involves a number of techniques to restore normal texture, flexibility, and function to affected tissues; decrease pain, knots, adhesions, and scar tissue; improve circulation; and optimize function of the soft tissue itself. In some cases, soft tissue therapy can feel good and relaxing, while at other times quite the opposite. Some therapies are passive, and others require active participation of the athlete. Some are done by highly trained professionals, and some can be self-administered, but ultimately the goal remains to decrease pain and increase function.

Techniques Administered by Others

Licensed massage therapists (LMT) employ many different therapeutic techniques. Clinicians might argue about theoretical differences between the approaches we are about to describe, but there is undoubtedly significant overlap in terms of the benefits, perhaps more than some practitioners would like to admit. Therefore, to a large extent, your choice comes down to what feels good and works for you.

In a muscle that has tightened up due to pain, weakness, or overuse, our goal is to decrease tension. Once we have been able to accomplish that release, we can more effectively strengthen the muscle, improve mobility and range of motion, and train the body to handle more load through that region with optimal movement strategies—all so that you're able to push hard on your runs.

Swedish Massage

The most prevalent technique is Swedish massage, which many runners swear by. While LMTs are often employed in spas or other places promoting relaxation, those same techniques can be valuable to athletes, as well.

Swedish massage can be relaxing and enjoyable for runners. It is typically not as intense as some other types of soft tissue therapy, making it suitable closer to race day. Swedish massage uses five techniques, all with the goal of encouraging circulation and loosening the tissue:

- Effleurage: Long strokes, always done toward the heart, to stimulate blood flow and venous return
- Petrissage: Deeper, kneading strokes
- Tapotement: Rhythmic tapping
- Friction: Deep, intense, localized technique for working on knots
- Vibration: A press and release technique

Active Release Technique (ART)

Active release technique, or ART, is a technique that has gained considerable momentum in the athletic community over the last 10 to 20 years. ART practitioners receive special training and require certification. ART is used by massage therapists, physical therapists, and chiropractors. The technique combines pressure applied by the practitioner to the affected area with movement using those muscles to address adhesions and scar tissue. Unlike Swedish massage, which generally addresses the whole body, ART is typically used to target specific muscles and related injuries or dysfunction. ART is an intense method and can result in temporary soreness afterward.

Myofascial Trigger Point Therapy

Another technique that may be of use for athletes is myofascial trigger point therapy, often referred to simply as trigger point therapy. Trigger points are knots, tender or tense areas of muscle that can negatively impact the function of the muscles. Trigger point therapists apply pressure to the affected areas and then move the muscle through a range of motion.

According to the David G. Simons Academy, which has taught trigger point therapy to therapists for decades, the goals of myofascial trigger point therapy are as follows:

- Improve blood circulation to the trigger zone
- Stretch the taut band
- Release the surrounding fasciae

Because of the intensity of this technique, it can be painful and result in soreness.

Instrument-Assisted Soft Tissue Mobilization

Instrument-assisted techniques—notably the Graston technique—are different from others used for runners. Graston, as an example, uses a special set of stainless steel tools on the muscles, coupled with massage. The technique works around adhesions and scar tissue, with the goal of stretching and relaxing the associated muscles to provide pain relief. With Graston and other soft tissue techniques, you can actually retrigger the body's inflammatory process to help surmount a plateau in healing. Aggressive work at, say, a tendon insertion can be an effective way to avoid more drastic and complex interventions like a platelet-rich plasma (PRP) or steroid injection. The intensity of instrument-assisted soft tissue mobilization can be adjusted by the practitioner's technique and according to the runner's tolerance, so while instrument-assisted techniques may seem intimidating, they aren't necessarily grueling.

Self-Massage Methods

While soft tissue work performed by a professional therapist is ideal in many ways, there are often obstacles, including finances and availability. Consequently, self-massage techniques have gained considerable popularity. The research on self-massage is still emerging, but there is reason for optimism with respect to its effectiveness in improving range of motion and muscle performance (Cheatham 2015).

Foam Rolling

Foam rollers were once a novelty but are now ubiquitous in gyms, physical therapy offices, and just about every runner's bedside or home gym. Foam rollers can be used on muscles from your calves to your hamstrings, from your quads to your lats. They can feel good (or, at times, not) and help promote circulation. They're inexpensive and can be used just about anywhere, making them a practical complement to other soft tissue work. In addition to foam rollers, items like tennis balls and lacrosse balls can be repurposed and used for self-massage.

Massage Guns

Massage guns are a relatively new tool that athletes can use to treat themselves. At first glance, you might mistake a massage gun for an electric drill, but thankfully it's used quite differently. Equipped with various heads and adjustable in intensity, a massage gun is handy and practical, and it may help ease the aches and pains associated with training and racing. Massage guns cannot easily reproduce long strokes, such as those used in Swedish massage, but they can be a good substitute for skilled hands when working out knots and adhesions. With these, the vibrations can distract your nervous system from the pain, thereby decreasing tensing, which often allows for a deeper release than what you can get from a foam roller alone. While most massage guns cost hundreds of dollars, the device is a onetime purchase that may save you multiple visits to a massage therapist.

Compression Boots

Another relatively new and popular tool in many athletes' soft tissue maintenance arsenal is a pneumatic compression set of devices commonly known as compression boots. Compression boots are worn over the legs and inflated to decrease swelling and reduce excess blood pooling in your legs. Proponents suggest that delayed onset muscle soreness (DOMS) decreases with their use. As with many newer devices, the scientific consensus on compression boots has yet to be reached, but there is reason for optimism. One study showed that ultramarathoners who used compression boots experienced equivalent muscle recovery to those who underwent massage therapy (Hoffman 2016).

Compression boots are not an insignificant investment, but they feel good and show promise when it comes to recovery. Many physical therapy offices offer them, providing a slightly less pricey option for runners who don't want to buy the technology outright. Compression boots do a good job replacing a long cool-down or active recovery because they prolong circulation to the extremities and promote blood flow and the uptake of lactic acid. It's pretty nice to be able to recline on the couch and have the boots do the work for you after an intense training session.

Timing of Soft Tissue Work

Determining when to get soft tissue work done can involve a few considerations. As we've outlined, some therapies are more intense than others and may therefore leave you sore in the days after. On the other hand, just as some runners tend to recover faster from a hard workout, some individuals are more (or less) affected by tissue work.

Because of the potential transient negative effects of a massage or other soft tissue work, it's generally not recommended that you get treated too close to race day. At the very least, be sure your therapist is aware of an upcoming race so they can adjust the intensity of their work. Similarly, because of the damaging inflammation and trauma to muscles after a hard race, it's typically not recommended to get work done in the first couple of days after a race. The postrace massages that you often see offered by race directors are a nice feature, but they should be gentle and have the goal of redistributing blood flow and relaxation rather than targeted, therapeutic work.

Conclusion

Regardless of which soft tissue therapies you use, appropriate treatment is a tool to help keep you running injury-free. Each has its advantages and disadvantages, with some being expensive and some requiring a trained professional, so it's worth experimenting to see what works for your body and your budget. Remember, decreasing tone (tension) in the nervous system helps the body let go, and everyone's nervous system works a little differently. Rather than taking your fast friend's opinion as gospel, it's important to experiment to figure out which techniques work best for your body.

PART II
BODY REGIONS

CHAPTER 5

Feet and Toes

In the next few chapters, we are going to cover injuries from the ground up, which means starting with the structures that literally connect with the ground and propel us forward when we run: our toes and feet. Foot and toe injuries in runners can come in all shapes and sizes, from blackened toenails to blisters, stress fractures to turf toe, bunions to arthritis. Although the cause of different foot and toe injuries varies, there are some overarching themes that injuries in this part of the body have in common.

Let's start by looking at the anatomy of the foot. Over 25 percent of the 206 bones of the adult human body are found in our feet (26 bones per foot, to be precise). That gives us a lot of moving parts. The foot is a unique structure—it is designed to be both highly flexible, to help us absorb the force of the ground when we land, and very rigid, to help us efficiently push off the ground and into the air as we run. Furthermore, our proprioception—which can loosely be defined as our awareness of where our body is in space, our sense of what type of terrain we are walking or running on, and our sense of balance and stability—comes through the sensory receptors in our feet.

Feet are, in a word, important. Yet for most of our lives, we cram our feet into shoes, depriving our body of proprioceptive input and, believe it or not, underutilizing an entire section of our brain. Moreover, modern footwear significantly hampers the foot's ability to splay (stretch out, with toes spread apart) when we land, which, over time, can increase the risk of developing bunions, neuromas, and other injuries and dysfunctions of the foot.

Research studies have shown a significant decrease in foot pliability and arch height in shoe wearers compared with population groups that are habitually barefoot (Franklin et al. 2015). This means that footwear negatively affects the two most basic functions of the foot: the ability of the foot to collapse when we land (because pliability helps with shock absorption and loading response) and the ability of the foot to tense and lock up when we push off (because the arch helps us efficiently transfer energy and momentum to drive ourselves forward). Furthermore, while diminished pliability and lower arches can cause foot problems, the effects of these deficiencies can also travel up the chain and ultimately affect the way we load joints at our knees, hips, and low back. You can see why it can be tricky to get to the root cause of an injury.

Are My Foot Problems Genetic?

We often hear complaints like "my doctor told me I have flat feet" or "my bunions are genetic." Let's clarify. While there absolutely are genetic factors contributing to your foot shape, genetics alone are not to blame for foot problems that develop. Ligamentous laxity, which is genetic, can predispose you to a flatter arch, but poor development of intrinsic foot muscles is also a controllable factor at play. Likewise, a wider foot or the anatomy of your hips can increase your chances of developing bunions, but another significant factor is years of wearing narrow shoes that limit the ability of your feet to splay when they land or of the big toe to operate when you push off.

Shoes and Running

Modern running shoes are designed to help conserve energy and increase efficiency—which, overall, are good things. However, this design isn't completely without consequence. Footwear changes the axis of rotation of your foot. Many shoes have a rocker bottom, designed to rock your foot forward and decrease the work of the foot and big toe during push-off. While this can be advantageous for improving your running economy and for rehabilitation, the con to this technology is that the big toe is not moving as much as it is designed to, which leads to a stiffening of the big toe joint. Over time, this stiffening can become permanent, strength and mobility are lost, and pain and inflammation often result.

It's also common for runners to prefer shoes that have a narrower fit, which gives a feeling of control and stability while running. However, the narrower the shoe, the less your toes can splay naturally when you land, leading to compression of the nerves, muscles, joints, and other structures of the foot.

While these issues might constitute an argument for choosing a wider, more minimalist running shoe, we are not advocating ditching shoes all together! Despite the problems that come with restricting the foot, we live in a modern world. Most people cannot realistically show up at their workplace barefoot, nor is it safe to forgo the protection of shoes in most outdoor situations. (It is not a good idea to run barefoot on concrete!) Instead, we tell our patients and athletes to seriously evaluate the footwear they choose when they aren't running. If you are running one to two hours a day, even in rocker-bottom or narrow shoes, permanent changes in foot structure will not occur as long as you are mindful of foot movement the other 22 to 23 hours of your day. This means choosing street shoes with a wider toe box, wearing high heels for only short periods of time, and going barefoot indoors whenever possible. It also means being proactive about foot strength and mobility. The exercises that we highlight in this chapter are intended to help you maintain proper foot strength and mobility in order to reduce or entirely prevent structural deformities from developing in your feet.

Orthotics

If you've gone to any running specialty store, in addition to the plethora of shoes available, you've probably also seen a wide selection of insoles. You may even run in a custom set of insoles made for you by your podiatrist.

Generally, we tend to discourage runners from relying on orthotics, because this caters to weaknesses and imbalances instead of addressing the root cause; it's a Band-Aid of sorts. However, in cases of acute inflammation or chronic injury, orthotics can play a key role in relieving an inflamed region, just as a cast can help to heal a broken arm. Also, if you've been running in orthotics for years, don't toss them out just yet! Your body has adapted to the support, so getting rid of them abruptly could cause injury. If you are considering transitioning out of orthotics, we recommend a gradual approach.

If you are struggling with an injury that may be more quickly healed with the help of orthotics, we highly recommend consulting your physical therapist or podiatrist.

Diagnosis

Because of the vast intricacies of the foot, we can't emphasize enough the importance of seeking professional help if you are dealing with a persistent foot or toe issue. Diagnosing your specific problem and its underlying cause without the specialized knowledge of a trained professional is challenging. That said, we will address a few of the most common conditions that affect runners' feet before we describe some foot and toe mobility exercises that help runners avoid these issues. Namely, we will address neuromas, bunions (hallux valgus), and stiff big toe (hallux rigidus).

Neuroma

A neuroma is the thickening and swelling of a nerve in the foot that causes painful burning, numbness, or tingling. This most commonly occurs between the third and fourth toes (metatarsals) and is referred to as *Morton's neuroma*.

Neuromas most often develop when the foot does not have adequate room to splay. When your foot is crammed into a shoe that is too tight, its joints are constricted, which can increase your risk of developing a neuroma. Additionally, repetitive pressure forces from your foot striking the ground can lead to neuroma. In particular, female runners who wear narrow-toed shoes or high heels to work and then go out and literally pound the pavement with their feet as they run are at increased risk of developing neuromas because of the excessive stress to the ball and metatarsal areas of the foot.

Typically, symptoms of a neuroma are exacerbated by wearing narrow shoes or repetitive pounding, and they can be alleviated by massage, stretching out the toes, or walking barefoot or in shoes with a wide toe box. Your doctor may also prescribe a small pad to insert into your shoe to alleviate pressure on a specific area.

Hallux Valgus (Bunion)

The etiology of bunions is similar to that of neuromas—namely, wearing shoes that are narrow or constrictive will increase your chances of developing a bunion. The development of a bunion can be even more connected to a runner's anatomy, specifically their foot structure, leading to complex compensations up and down the chain. Foot width plays a big role in the development of a bunion, as does hip anatomy.

If your thigh bone sits at a certain angle in your hip socket (rotated backward, or femoral retroversion), you are prone to compensating with a toe-out gait pattern that puts stress on the big toe and changes the line of push-off, or lever arm, from straight to angled (figure 5.1). A similar effect can result from cramming your foot into a shoe that is too small; it can change the lever from which your big toe pushes off the ground. Over time, this movement pattern can lead to structural changes in the bones of the foot—the development of hallux valgus, or a bunion.

Symptoms of a bunion include having a big toe that points inward instead of straight (see figure 5.2), swelling on the outside of your toe, and pain

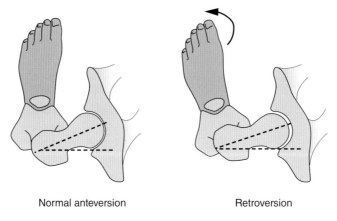

Normal anteversion   Retroversion

Figure 5.1   Retroversion contributes to the development of a toe-out bunion.

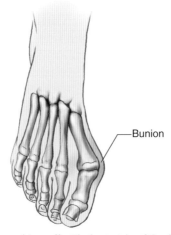

—Bunion

Figure 5.2   Over time, reliance on pushing off with the inside of the foot instead of with big toe extensors can lead to anatomical changes.

with push-off. Not all bunions are painful, and you may very well be able to proceed with your running and training with this deformity without issue. However, while your toes might feel okay, a bunion can be a driving factor for other injuries. Because bunions are often linked to a toe-out gait pattern, this can put more stress on the arch of your foot and the inside of your knee, and it may even affect your hip and low back.

Hallux Rigidus (Stiff Big Toe, Big Toe Arthritis, or Turf Toe)

Similar to a bunion, hallux rigidus—also referred to as *stiff big toe*, *big toe arthritis*, or *turf toe*—affects the big toe. The difference is that instead of the inward angle of your big toe increasing, you begin to lose the ability to bend the big toe due to a stiffening of the joint capsule, which can affect your ability to push off when you walk and run. Over time, compensations can cause hallux rigidus to turn into hallux valgus (bunion). Since you aren't able to propel off your big toe, the foot will start to rotate inward slightly, causing the lever of push-off to come from the inside of the foot. Hallux rigidus can be caused by compensations that follow an acute strain of the big toe or by excessive load on the joint stemming from similar imbalances (Camasta 1996; Jafary 2020).

Case Study: Nora

Nora presents to physical therapy with pain in her big toe. She reports that the pain is definitely worse with running, but it seems aggravated just from walking around the city. She has been trying to wear her sneakers for walking instead of her normal boots, but she's still struggling to overcome the toe pain.

Observation: Nora wears narrow sneakers that don't allow her foot to splay when landing, and she spends a lot of her time in boots that also restrict her toe mobility. Nora also exhibits a toe-out gait pattern, which puts excessive load on her first MTP joint (the joint connecting the big toe to the foot bone), and she is unable to isolate any big toe movement. Nora's big toe is slightly swollen laterally and is very mildly angled inward. She is also extremely restricted in her big toe flexion and extension.

Diagnosis: Hallux rigidus and valgus; not yet a bunion but headed that way.

Treatment: Treatment for Nora consists of joint mobilization for her big toe and all of her foot, specifically distraction and flexion/extension, performed by her physical therapist. Nora is educated on the importance of wearing wider footwear when on her feet for a prolonged time (such as commuting by walking) and is given strengthening exercises for her big toe and her arch (lift, spread, reach; big toe extension). Kinesiology tape is used to guide the toe medially and provide Nora with tactical feedback for pushing off through her toe and medial arch. Nora also intermittently uses a toe spacer to help promote toe splaying when she walks. These interventions help her symptoms resolve, and she continues to keep up with toe stretching and careful choice of footwear to avoid developing a bunion.

Treatment and Prevention

When it comes to foot and toe injuries, two themes emerge: These injuries are instigated either by a foot that has grown stiff due to too much time crammed into a narrow or too-small shoe or by a foot that, over time, has grown weak, again because of too much time in a shoe. These themes are not mutually exclusive; more often than not, a foot can exhibit a combination of stiffness and weakness, leading to increased risk of injury.

The first line of defense is mindfulness of footwear, both when you are running and when you are not. Here are a few pointers:

- If you are experiencing pain or inflammation in the big toe, a shoe with an increased rocker bottom will lessen the workload of that toe, which can help. But remember, this is a Band-Aid approach, so definitely read on in the next section about restorative exercises!

- A good indicator for when to transition out of this type of shoe comes from symptoms of pain or swelling; once you are able to walk without pain or notice a significant decrease in inflammation, you can begin to transition out of this type of supportive footwear. We recommend a gradual transition, going on short walks in flatter or less supportive shoes and slowly increasing the minutes per day that you are on your feet in those non-rocker footwear. Make sure you have wiggle room for your toes. For running shoes, we usually recommend going up a half or sometimes even a full size from what you wear in your normal everyday shoes.

- When you're not running, follow this general rule: Barefoot is better. Try to spend most of your time walking around your house barefoot instead of in shoes (even slippers), unless you are dealing with an acute injury or pain.

- Limit the amount of time you spend in pointy-toed shoes, shoes with a narrow toe box (i.e., shoes that prohibit you from lifting up your toes or spreading them apart), high heels, boots, or flip-flops. While it is unrealistic to insist that runners *never* wear these, try to save them for infrequent occasions. If you must wear restrictive shoes at a formal event or at work, commute in comfy shoes and switch over when you arrive. If that's not possible, try to make sure you follow up a day spent in fashion shoes or flip-flops with a set of foot maintenance exercises like the ones described in this chapter.

The second line of defense against foot and toe problems is toe exercises designed to promote increased mobility and strength in the toes and arch.

Splay Your Feet

This exercise is easy to understand but often challenging to execute. Start by lifting your toes while keeping the rest of your foot flat on the ground. Spread your toes apart as far as possible (figure 5.3*a*), and then push them back down into the ground, with emphasis on the distal portion of your big toe extending firmly into the ground, not curling under (figure 5.3*b*). The focus is on toe disassociation, intrinsic activation, and mobilization of the arch.

You might be asking, "Why am I doing this?" What we are looking for is the ability to move our toes separately from each other while actively engaging and strengthening our arch. If you have a very stiff foot or arch, this is a great beginning exercise. We recommend starting with both feet together and progressing to one foot at a time.

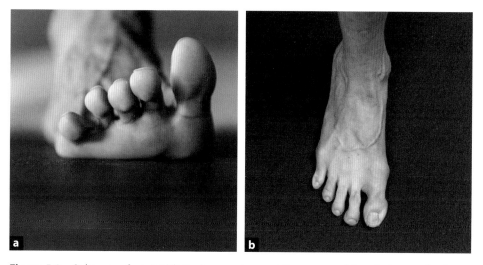

Figure 5.3   Splay your feet: *(a)* lift the toes and spread them apart; *(b)* push the toes back into the ground.

Toe Yoga

This is another exercise that is harder than it looks. Start with your foot flat on the ground. Lift your big toe while the little toes push down (figure 5.4a). Then lift the little toes while the big toe pushes down (figure 5.4b). Alternate. If you're struggling, start with two feet and progress to one foot at a time.

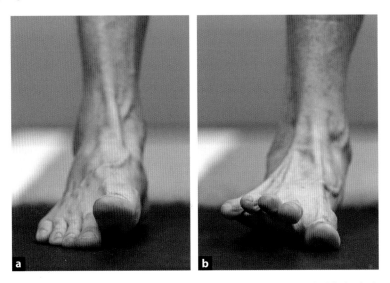

Figure 5.4   Toe yoga: (a) lift the big toe and push the little toes down; (b) lift the little toes and push the big toe down.

Active Assisted Range of Motion for Toes

If splaying your feet and toe yoga are too challenging, start with this simpler exercise. Sit in a chair or on the ground (whatever's comfortable) and, using your hands, move your toes individually, one at a time (figure 5.5*a* and figure 5.9*b*). You can apply some distraction, meaning you are bracing the ball of your foot with one hand while pulling the toe away from your body while bending the toe back and forth. Some cracks and pops are totally OK; in fact, they are a good sign! Keep trying the other two exercises, however, because eventually you'll see movement sans hands!

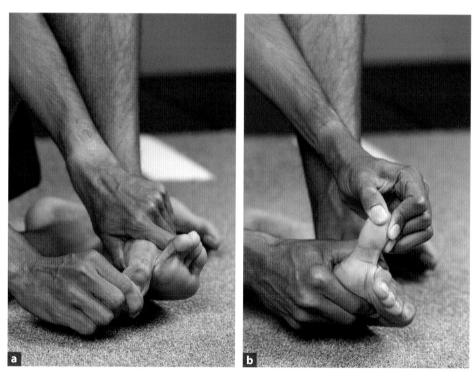

Figure 5.5   Active assisted range of motion for toes: *(a)* start position to move big toe; *(b)* finish position when moving big toe.

Arch Stretch

Stand with one foot in front of you, flat on the ground. Move that same knee forward and inward over your toes (imagine a diagonal line at an approximately 45-degree angle) to facilitate flattening and stretching the arch of the foot (figure 5.6).

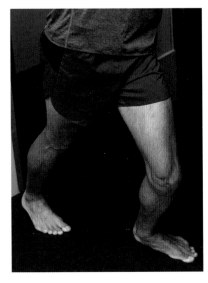

Figure 5.6   Arch stretch.

Pronation Driver

The pronation driver is similar to the arch stretch, but the goal is to collapse the arch downward and facilitate end-range pronation, which is particularly useful if you have a rigid foot. You'll start the same way as with the arch stretch (figure 5.6); the goal this time is a dynamic stretch in which you are working to collapse the arch downward in order to increase the foot's ability to pronate. Instead of holding the stretch, drive the knee forward (heel to toe) and then relax back slightly, aiming to get more and more pronation through the arch with each rep. It can be helpful to use your body weight to facilitate an increased stretch. For bonus points, add a roll through the big toe at the end of the stretch.

Arch Activation: Supination Driver and Short Foot

These two exercises can be used to activate your arch, which is useful if you have a more hypermobile or flat foot. The first exercise is a supination driver. The opposite of the pronation driver, this involves stepping into internal rotation to engage the arch with external rotation of the femur, tibia, and midfoot (figure 5.7). Start by standing on one foot. With your other foot, step into a T shape, bringing the leg around (toes first) and in front. With your hands on your hips, rotate your pelvis toward the stance leg and note your femur, tibia, and arch engaging and lifting. Make sure you keep your big toe pressed into the ground.

The short foot exercise involves doming the arch by pressing other parts of the foot into the ground. Standing on one leg, connect your big toe, pinky toe, and heel with the ground by pressing firmly down. Then lift your arch off the ground.

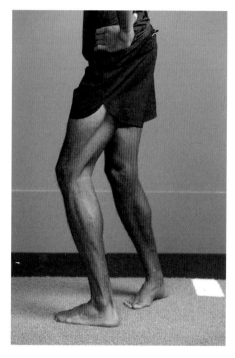

Figure 5.7 Arch activation: supination driver.

Three-Way Balance Driver

A general balance exercise, the three-way balance driver challenges your balance, proprioception, and stability with multidirectional movement. It also hones your ability to react to different external factors you'll encounter in your environment, such as running on uneven surfaces or navigating curbs. This exercise builds strength and resilience through the ankle ligaments and can help build resistance to ankle sprains (discussed more in chapter 6).

Stand on an unstable surface. A foam pad, couch cushion, carpet, or even yoga mat can work. Balancing on one leg, start by reaching the other foot forward, then backward, tapping your toe softly in each direction (figure 5.8*a* and 5.8*b*). Begin with a small range; as you get stronger you can progress by trying to reach farther. Next, tap your foot from side to side (across your body) (figure 5.8*c* and 5.8*d*). The same idea applies: Start with a small range and progress to a bigger movement. Finally, you'll twist in, making a T shape with your feet (internal rotation), and out, making an L shape with your feet (figure 5.8*e* and 5.8*f*). When you're ready to progress to a more advanced unstable surface, you can use a balance-training half ball.

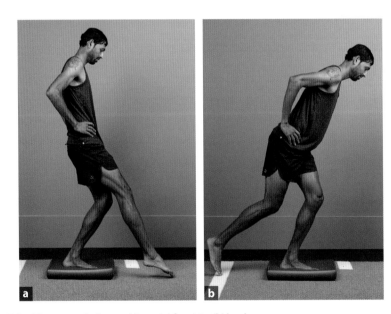

Figure 5.8 Three-way balance driver: *(a)* front to *(b)* back.

Three-way balance driver learned from Gray Institute°, GrayInstitute.com.

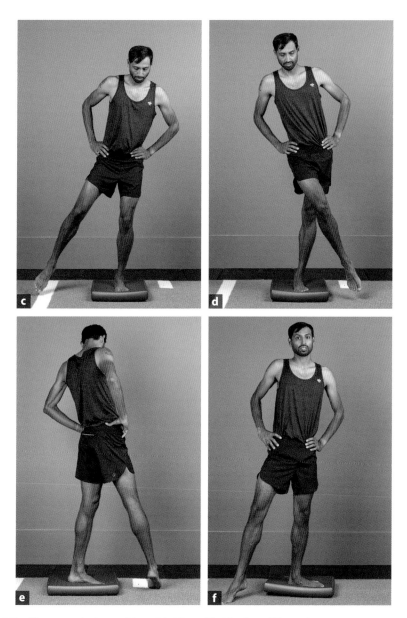

Figure 5.8   Three-way balance driver: *(c)* side to *(d)* side; *(e and f)* rotation.

Toe Separators

This last one isn't an exercise, but rather a product. If you've ever had a pedicure, you already know what toe separators are: They're the little foam or soft plastic devices that you stick between your toes in order to keep them apart. We recommend getting silicone ones that have one flat edge so they're easier to walk in. Wear them as long as you can tolerate when you are barefoot in your home.

Conclusion

While toe and foot injuries come in all shapes and sizes, understanding some of the common themes can be useful for runners when treating and preventing toe and foot problems. Of course, none of the exercises and tips we've presented can take the place of an evaluation by a professional, so if you are having pain, swelling, or discomfort in the toes or feet, please seek treatment from a physical therapist, podiatrist, or orthopedist.

CHAPTER 6

Ankles

It's happened to the best of us: a misstep off a curb while on a run, an errant step into a pothole, or a trip over a hidden tree root. The classic inward roll or twist of the ankle, the sudden gasp of pain. At this point, as we hobble back to our apartment, house, or car, we'll tell anyone who asks: "I twisted my ankle." It could be a sprain, strain, or even fracture, but what most runners immediately want to know is *should I stop running*?

It depends.

To understand an ankle injury, we first need to understand how the ankle is designed to work. Due to the anatomy of the bones in the ankle joint, the ankle is designed to move in all three planes of motion (front to back, side to side, and rotationally; described in chapter 1). At the ankle, the six movements are referred to as dorsiflexion and plantar flexion (moving the ankle up and down, like pumping a gas pedal), inversion and eversion (moving the ankle in and out), and pronation and supination (the rotational response of the ankle to landing and pushing off). These movements are made up of a combination of movement at your subtalar joint, calcaneus, and foot and make up the landing and push-off phases of gait (figure 6.1*a* and figure 6.1*b*). All of this is to say, the ankle is a complex part of your body. This joint is designed for mobility, as opposed to other joints, such as the lower back and knee, which are built for stability. Just like the foot, the

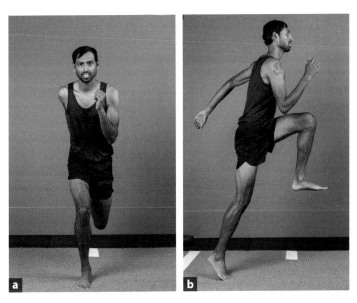

Figure 6.1 *(a)* Running landing: pronation, dorsiflexion, eversion. *(b)* Running push-off: supination, plantar flexion, inversion.

ankle plays an integral roll in shock absorption while landing and as a rigid lever for efficient energy transfer in push-off.

In addition to its bones being designed for mobility, the ankle has ligaments that are critical to our awareness of where our bodies are in space—a sense known as *proprioception*. In fact, compared to other joints in the body, ankle proprioception has been shown to be the most important indicator of sports performance (Han et al. 2015). Imagine your proprioceptive sense as a tiny brain that lives in your ankles. When your feet hit the ground, the ligaments in your ankles send signals to your (real) brain to tell you the type of surface you are landing on and where your body is in relationship to your surroundings. All this signaling helps you to maintain balance and stability throughout your entire body. However, when our ankle ligaments are damaged, we lose this sense of proprioception. If the damage is severe enough, continuing to run with this reduced sense of proprioception can be detrimental. Not only will running continue to place stress on the damaged tendons and ligaments of the ankle, but the risk of reinjury is greater because of the lack of proprioception (Han et al. 2015). With the ankle, it's a slippery slope—continuing to run on a small ankle tweak can turn into a season-ending injury. Don't go down that slope!

Diagnosis

When you roll your ankle, there are generally two structures that you can injure: ligaments and tendons. A severe ankle sprain can sometimes even lead to an avulsion fracture of the ankle bone, meaning that the force is so strong that instead of the ankle ligaments or tendons stretching and tearing, a piece of the bone actually breaks off. In the following sections, we outline the similarities and differences between an injury to the ligaments and to the tendons in your ankle.

Ligament Injury (Ankle Sprain)

After you roll your ankle, any swelling, bruising, or tenderness indicates that you likely have an ankle sprain. A sprain means that the ligaments (which, if you remember, connect bone to bone) that stabilize the ankle and control movement have been overstretched or sometimes even slightly torn. Depending on the severity of your injury, the amount of time you'll need to recover can range from a couple of days to several months.

The first phase of healing involves the growth of scar tissue, or immature collagen fibers. These fibers do not receive the same proprioceptive input as the undamaged ligaments, so full proprioception can be tricky to regain. This etiology explains why, if not properly rehabilitated, ankle sprains can become a recurring issue. Once the ankle loses its "brain," or sense of awareness in space, it's only a matter of time until another misplaced footstep causes it to reroll.

What Increases My Chances of an Ankle Injury?

Besides genetics and prior sprains, other factors that can increase your risk of ankle injury include weakness in your core, hips, ankles, and arches. Core and hip weakness can increase dynamic, uncontrolled pronation in landing, which puts more stress on the inside of the foot. Ankle and arch weakness can also contribute to this uncontrolled pronation, putting more stress on the ankle joint.

Alternatively, a more supinated (outward) gait pattern can put you at greater risk of rolling an ankle on a run because you are landing on the outside of your foot, which has less ability to load or absorb shock. Limited pronation has been found to significantly increase your chance of an ankle sprain injury (Colapietro et al. 2020). You need your feet to follow the Goldilocks principle: You don't want a foot that is too rigid or too mobile but a foot that is right in between.

Consequently, a prior insufficiently rehabbed ankle sprain can predict future ankle sprains. However, certain genetic factors can play a role in your ankle sprain likelihood, too. Too much ligamentous stiffness or laxity—which comes from the length and width of your tendons and the strength of their collagen fibers, all of which you inherited—can affect your susceptibility to ankle sprains. Your innate proprioceptive skill, or coordination, can factor in, too.

Tendon Injury

Remember the section on ligaments in chapter 1? Once the integrity of the ligament is lost, it is very hard to regain. Therefore, chronic ankle sprains can lead to ligamentous laxity, which can cause excessive movement of the foot in walking and running. Too much foot movement can, in turn, cause increased torque on the ligaments and tendons on either side of the foot and ankle, placing extra stress on surrounding muscles and tendons—which can ultimately lead to a secondary or overuse ankle injury like peroneal or posterior tibial tendinitis.

Unlike an acute ankle sprain, an overuse injury has a more gradual onset. You may start off feeling a little bit of discomfort in your ankle at the end of a run, and that discomfort may begin to worsen over time. Because a muscle group is usually involved, symptoms may extend up into the leg or down into the foot.

Alternatively, an acute strain to a tendon (remember, tendons connect muscle to bone) can present similarly to an ankle sprain, with an immediate feeling of "ouch!" The differences between an acute tendon strain and an acute ligament sprain are minor, and the differences in rehabilitation are equally minor; a professional can help you distinguish between the two. A tendon strain, which can feel like a ligament strain, is an acute injury (i.e., it's sudden), whereas tendinitis is a chronic (i.e., overuse) injury.

Tendinitis Versus Tendinosis

Tendons can easily fall victim to acute (strain) or overuse (tendinitis) injuries. In the latter case, tendons in the ankle can also progress from tendinitis to tendinosis. Distinguishing between these two injuries often comes down to time. In a clinical setting (if, for example, you are evaluated by a physical therapist) you will be asked how long you've been experiencing symptoms. If the duration has been for less than six weeks, they will probably diagnose you with tendinitis—i.e., inflammation of the tendon caused by microtears that happen due to acute overloading of the tendon by forces that are too heavy, too sudden, or too demanding. Over time, however, these microtears can cause more substantial tissue degeneration, as well as structural changes in the anatomy of the tendon or heel bone on which the tendon inserts (Bass 2012). Therefore, if your symptoms have lasted longer than six weeks, you will probably be diagnosed with tendinosis.

Tendinosis is the degeneration of the tendon's collagen in response to chronic overuse. Instead of becoming inflamed as the result of overload, the tendon thickens and increases in stiffness. Misaligned, immature collagen fibers start to build up. Instead of a strong, parallel alignment that facilitates strength with load-bearing, the fibers are disorganized and not as structurally sound (Asplund and Best 2013). The proprioceptive "brain" won't work as well, and the ankle is less resilient to a future misstep, so your chance of injury increases.

Case Study: Imani

Imani presents with lateral ankle pain that began after a trail run. Imani does not recall an acute roll of her ankle, but she is having a lot of pain on the outside of her foot when walking and reports that she can't walk without a limp.

Extra stress on the outside of a foot for someone who is more pronated, or extra stress on the inside of a foot for someone who is more supinated, can be problematic. Remember, the body adapts to the load placed on it, so the body can get very strong at its compensations. Therefore, changing the movement (and stress) pattern too quickly can also cause irritation and inflammation.

Observation: Imani presents with a very rigid gait. She is not letting her arch roll in when she walks, and she is very guarded. She feels tenderness when the physical therapist palpates the outside of her ankle, and her movement is restricted in both eversion and inversion.

Diagnosis: Acute peroneal tendinitis.

Treatment: Imani's physical therapist helps to mobilize the peroneal tendon and performs soft tissue work on the peroneal muscle belly and joint mobilizations to the calcaneus. Imani is given exercises for eccentric loading of lateral ankle (described shortly), plus inversion and eversion banded ankle exercises. Once she is pain-free, Imani performs pronation driver exercises and works her way toward "reeducating" her ankle on proper gait.

Treatment and Prevention

As you may expect, the first step to treating an ankle injury is distinguishing what type of injury you have. If you are uncertain or are experiencing acute pain, swelling, and discomfort with weight-bearing, we strongly recommend that you get checked out by a doctor to rule out a fracture or severe sprain or tear that may require complete immobilization. However, if you are confident in your diagnosis based on the material described thus far, read on.

Sprain or Strain

If what you are experiencing is indeed an acute ankle sprain or strain, pause for a second before you reach for the bag of ice or frozen peas. Ice has its place but should be used sparingly; we recommend icing for no more than 10 minutes and doing so only within the first six hours of injury. The reason is that in reducing inflammation, ice can actually delay the body's natural healing process by restricting blood flow to an injured area (Mirkin 2020). Elevation and compression, on the other hand, are often the best tools in the immediate aftermath of an acute ankle sprain or strain and can be used more liberally. Both help to reduce swelling, and compression has the added benefit of promoting blood flow to the region.

While the ligaments and tendons are healing, limit movement and stress on the foot—which, yes, means taking a break from running. However, while too much movement can worsen symptoms or the injury itself, complete immobility is often not the answer either. Immobility leads to decreased blood flow to the area, which can delay healing and increase pain. The surrounding muscles can begin to atrophy, and excess scar tissue can begin to form. Therefore, while a good rule of thumb is to avoid any movement that causes pain, gentle active or active-assisted range of motion exercises can often be performed without pain and can promote healing to the damaged tissues. Active-assisted movements mean that you are using either your own hands or a band to move the joint through more range than you could do with voluntary muscle engagement without causing pain (partially assisted, partially your own body doing the work) to work on strength and mobility without aggravating the injured area.

We recommend starting with simple ankle circles and ankle inversion, eversion, plantar flexion, and dorsiflexion within the pain-free range. Gradually progress to the 3D banded strength, detailed later in this chapter, and balance taps, part of the three-way balance driver described in chapter 5. This is a great starting place in rehabbing the ankle and building resilience to decrease future injury risk.

Ankle Braces

Given that most people must walk at least a little bit in their day-to-day lives, ankle braces can help someone suffering from an ankle strain by providing artificial support to the ankle externally in order to decrease the work required by the injured area. However, this short-term solution should not be used as a permanent fix; six to eight weeks is typically the maximum time someone should wear a brace. As the ankle tendon and ligaments are healing, you can gradually wean yourself off the brace by going on short, and later longer, walks without the brace. Then, provided you experience no increases in pain, you can start with a short run without the brace and gradually progress from there.

The Bauerfeind Sports Ankle Support is a great brace because it has both a soft, compressive component that can help with swelling and a more stable support from the band that doesn't limit movement as much as a full boot or rigid brace.

Shoe Assistance

If you are dealing with a chronic or overuse ankle injury, you probably know that rest alone is not the answer. That said, modifications are necessary. If you are dealing with medial ankle tendinitis (sometimes called *posterior tibial tendinitis*), wearing a shoe or insole with some medial support (i.e., pronation control) can help to off-load pressure in the afflicted area and allow the inflamed structures to calm down. Then, to prevent it from recurring, proper foot, ankle, and hip strengthening protocols—as prescribed by a physical therapist—can be used to address the root of the problem. Alternatively, lateral ankle stress (peroneal tendinitis) may benefit from a more neutral cushioned shoe or insert that aids in loading the inside of the foot more, which helps to decrease stress on the outer ankle. No matter which type of tendinitis you have, you'll benefit from running on a smooth, flat surface and avoiding uneven surfaces, trails, or hills, all of which increase the load on the affected ankle structures.

Eccentrics

This method of treatment is tried and true for tendon pathology, whether you're dealing with a strain, tendinitis, or tendinosis. Remember, eccentric muscle contraction is the slow, controlled lengthening of a muscle—this generates the most amount of power or force through muscle fibers. Eccentric exercises are thought of as the gold standard for tendon rehabilitation because these types of exercises help to realign collagen fibers, strengthen the muscle, and promote blood flow to the tissue. One example of an eccentric exercise for ankle rehabilitation is the slow, controlled lowering of the ankle into inversion or eversion (figure 6.2a-d). You can use a resistance band to

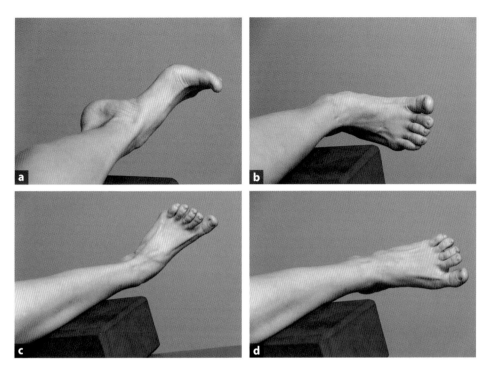

Figure 6.2   Eccentric ankle exercise: *(a-b)* inversion; *(c-d)* eversion.

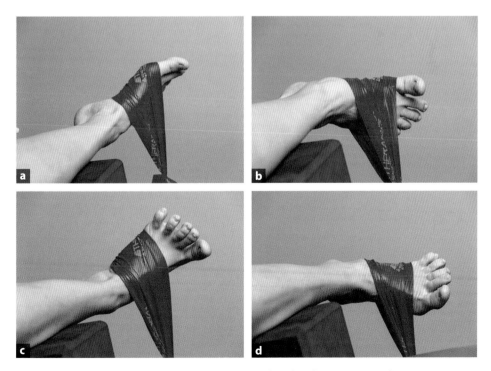

Figure 6.3   Eccentric ankle exercise with resistance band: *(a-b)* inversion; *(c-d)* eversion.

make this more challenging by facilitating an eccentric contraction with resistance (figure 6.3a-d).

The magic of eccentrics lies in the slow, controlled lengthening of the tissue; this is a powerful way to both promote blood flow and to work on realigning the damaged muscle or collagen fibers. One thing to watch out for, though, is introducing these movements too early in rehabilitation, before the tendon has had enough time to adequately heal from its initial trauma. We recommend waiting eight weeks after the initial injury to begin these exercises, although a professional may be able to guide you to incorporate eccentric activity earlier.

Mobility Exercises

Before you get too deep into ankle strengthening, make sure you've restored functional range of motion to the ankle joint. The reason is that otherwise you'll be limited in how much you can functionally strengthen a muscle or joint that isn't able to move through the full range of motion.

Soft Tissue Mobilization

We recommend starting with soft tissue mobilization (a fancy term for self-massage) to loosen up the muscles and soft tissues around the ankle joint before getting into dynamic mobilization. A foam roller is a great tool to start with. For the calf specifically, a lacrosse ball can work well to dig a little deeper than a foam roller (if you can tolerate it!). Start by sitting on the floor with your legs extended in front of you, toes pointed to the ceiling. Press the muscle with the foam roller or lacrosse ball right above the Achilles and work your way up little by little, incorporating ankle pumps up and down or circles with your foot for active release. Next, we recommend targeting both the lateral and medial ankle—your peroneal muscles and your posterior tibialis—in a similar fashion. Work the foam roller or lacrosse ball up the ankle along the inside of the shin bone (posterior tibialis; figure 6.4) as well as laterally along your fibula, using the same active release techniques.

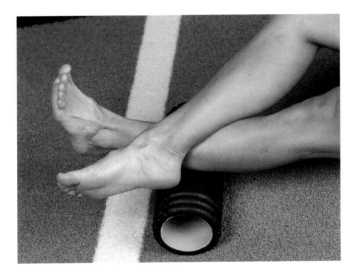

Figure 6.4 Foam rolling the calf.

Ankle Massage

You can also use your hands to massage around the two ankle bones (medial and lateral malleolus); sometimes the tendon in the space between the ankle bone and the Achilles tendon can get restricted as it wraps around the ankle bone. Try slowly moving your thumbs along this area while pressing down. You can also work directly along either side of the Achilles tendon as you move your ankle up and down. These techniques work to improve tissue mobility and increase dorsiflexion, inversion, and eversion range of motion.

3D Calf Stretch

Finally, one more mobility exercise is the 3D calf stretch (figure 6.5). Brace two hands on a wall and stagger your stance so your nonworking leg is in front of you. Lean forward slightly. Lift the knee of the non-working leg; you will use this leg as a driver to mobilize the rear lower leg. Move the working calf in all three planes of motion—front to back (figure 6.5*a*), side to side (figure 6.5, *b* and *c*), and twisting in and out (figure 6.5, *d* and *e*)—leading with your hips and using the non-working leg as a driver. Never push to the point of pain or discomfort, instead aiming for a productive stretch.

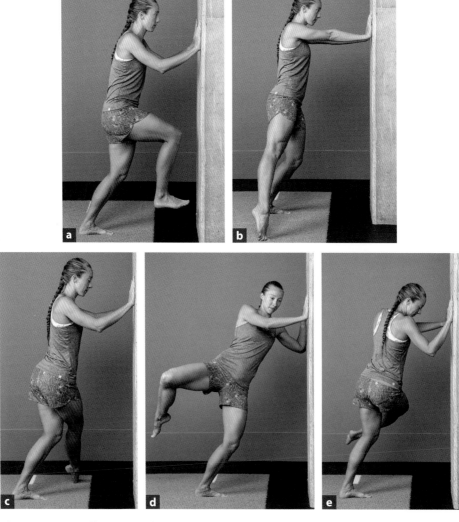

Figure 6.5   3D calf stretch: *(a)* front to back; *(b* and *c)* side to side; *(d* and *e)* rotation. 3D calf stretch learned from Gray Institute®, GrayInstitute.com.

Stability Exercises

Given our earlier discussion of the role of the ankle brain in our ability to move through space, stability and balance retraining are key components of ankle rehabilitation. Here are a few of our favorite exercises for increasing the triplanar dynamic strength of your ankle. Just remember that if you are coming back from an acute ankle injury, never push through pain or discomfort with any of these exercises.

For general strengthening, exercises such as lateral taps or monster walks, single-leg posterior taps, lateral step-ups or hip drops, plyometrics, double-leg hops, side-to-side hops, speed skaters, and running drills are good choices.

3D Banded Strength Exercises

Inversion: Sit with your legs extended and feet unsupported (for example, off the side of your couch or bed). Loop a resistance band around your ankle. Cross your other leg over the working leg, looping the band around this foot to anchor the band. The resistance should be lateral. Bring the working foot down and inward (figure 6.6*a*). You should feel the muscles on the inside of the ankle tense. Slowly, and with control, return the ankle back to neutral resting position.

Eversion: Sit with both legs extended. Loop the band around the non-working foot so the resistance is pulling medially. Bring the foot up and out to the same side (figure 6.6*b*). You should feel your outer shin muscles working after a few reps. Control the ankle as you return to neutral. Perform 2 or 3 sets of 10 repetitions or to tolerance.

Plantar flexion: Push the foot away from you like you are pumping a gas pedal (figure 6.6*c*). Again, control the return to neutral.

Dorsiflexion: Pull your foot toward you while the band is anchored away from you (figure 6.6*d*), and then return to neutral with control.

If you can perform all 3D banded strength exercises pain-free, progress to the following exercises from chapter 5: three-way balance driver, pronation driver, and supination driver.

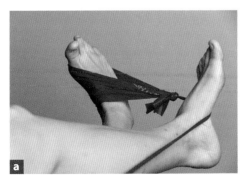 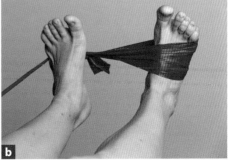

Figure 6.6   3D banded strength exercises: *(a)* inversion; *(b)* eversion.

(continued)

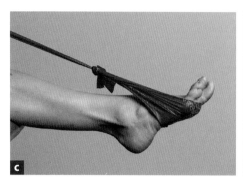 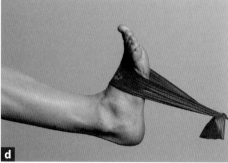

Figure 6.6 3D banded strength exercises: *(c)* plantar flexion; *(d)* dorsiflexion.

Training Considerations

As with every injury discussed in this book, if you are experiencing ankle pain, we highly recommend seeking out a medical professional for an evaluation and treatment plan. If you choose to keep running through an ankle injury, here are a few tips to keep in mind, based on everything we've discussed thus far:

- Don't rely on ice. Consistently treating your ankle with ice might make it feel better temporarily, but it will only delay the healing process. Stick with compression and elevation in the initial stages of healing and decrease the stress on your ankle and foot until you can begin active rehabilitation.

- An ankle brace can help to decrease the stabilization work of the ligaments and tendons as they are healing, but it can also affect your running form, stride length, and overall economy. An ankle brace should not be used as a long-term fix.

- Footwear—namely a temporary insole or stability shoe—can sometimes do the trick to limit the work of the inside of the ankle, which can allow the area to heal while you stay active. Likewise, if you have outer-ankle pain, a more neutral shoe can promote pronation, helping to decrease the force on the outside of your ankle with landing. Having the right pair of sneakers can also help to reduce your chance of ankle injury. This is where seeking out an expert shoe fit at a running specialty store is one of the best investments you can make.

- Time spent on strength, balance, foam rolling, and stretching helps to reduce the load and promote blood flow to the injured areas.

- Smooth, flat surfaces are ideal for decreasing the torque of the ankle while you are still injured. On the other hand, if you are healthy, incorporating dirt or trail running can help to strengthen the ankle to prevent injury and build resilience to future injuries.

Conclusion

As you've probably realized, ankles are pretty complicated, and there are lots of different injury possibilities that can affect this joint. Be wary of running through an ankle injury, because it can very quickly lead to a second injury due to gait and stride modifications that are hard to self-regulate. If you are unsure what might be wrong with your ankle, see your doctor or physical therapist as soon as possible.

CHAPTER 7

Knees

As a runner, you won't be surprised to learn that knee injuries are the most common area of injury that runners face (Van Gent et al. 2007). However, what we often term *knee injury* simply refers to where the runner feels pain; the knee itself is rarely the culprit.

Many health care professionals advise runners to avoid or cut back on running to "save their knees." While there is some research correlating long-distance running to increased risk of knee osteoarthritis, we subscribe to the mantra that "it's never the knee's fault." If proper training strategy, strength, and biomechanics are maintained, your knees should experience very little overload while running.

Let's first take a look at the anatomy of the knee joint (figure 7.1). The knee joint is composed of the femur up top, patella (kneecap) in the middle, and tibia on the bottom. The quadriceps muscles on top work to extend or straighten the knee. The quadriceps muscles attach to the patella via the quadriceps tendon, and the patella attaches to the tibia via the patellar ligament. This system works like a pulley for efficient transfer of energy from upper to lower leg. Behind the knee, the hamstring muscles work to flex or bend the knee. The meniscus, a thick pad of cartilage, sits between the femur and tibia; its main role is to absorb shock and impact on the knee and facilitate smooth motion as the knee bends back and forth and rotates in and out. Finally, the knee is surrounded by a thick retinaculum, or connective tissue, that functions to stabilize the knee.

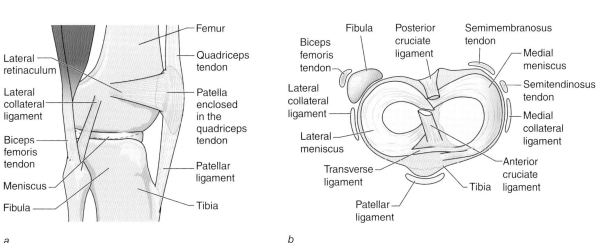

a

b

Figure 7.1 Knee joint: *(a)* side view and *(b)* top view.

Compared to the hip or the ankle, the knee is a relatively simple joint designed primarily for flexion and extension, or bending back and forth. While a small amount of internal and external rotation occurs at the knee, primarily to load and unload the joint, the joints above and below the knee—the hip and the ankle—have a much greater capacity for rotational forces. Consequently, restrictions in the hip or the ankle can often lead to excessive torque, movement, and force through the knee joint and are often the main drivers of knee pain.

Gait Cycle

Before we get into the causes of and solutions to knee pain, we first must understand how the knee functions when we run.

When a runner lands on the ground, the leg rotates inward (in a controlled manner) to properly absorb shock. The foot pronates down and inward, and then the tibia and femur both internally rotate. When a runner pushes off, the reverse happens: The femur and tibia externally rotate, and then the foot supinates, becoming a rigid lever for powerful and efficient forward propulsion. Because of their structure, the hip and ankle are more suited to both load and transfer rotational forces. If rotation is lost at the hip or the ankle, the knee gets "stuck" in the middle and must try to perform the rotation that the hip or ankle can no longer do in order for you to keep running. But remember, the knee doesn't want to rotate very much! So this added "forced" rotation is what often irritates the knee and causes injury.

The knee joint is designed to maintain some degree of flexion throughout the running gait cycle (figure 7.2). This helps with load distribution across the knee and is also a sign that both anterior (quads) and posterior (glutes and hamstrings) chain muscles are working in balance during gait. The quad muscles are designed to primarily function eccentrically in running, meaning they are able to decelerate movement and help with shock absorption on landing. The glutes, meanwhile, work as the power driver, propelling you forward.

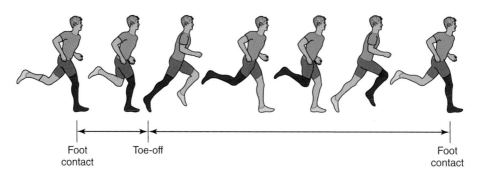

Foot contact   Toe-off   Foot contact

Figure 7.2   Gait cycle.

Tightness in the quadriceps muscles can make it hard to maintain knee flexion, because the quads pull the knee into extension. Tightness in the quads and hip flexors can also limit hip extension, making it harder for the glutes to fire. When the glutes aren't firing, the quads often wind up over-compensating. When the quadriceps are tight or overworking, the muscles pull the patella into the joint and limit its ability to glide smoothly back and forth. This increases compressive forces at the knee joint. This tightness can also contribute to overstriding, i.e., landing with the foot in front of you rather than beneath you, which causes increased loading on the knee on landing.

Weakness in the glutes or hamstrings can lead to overworking the quads in running, again resulting in greater force transfer through the knee. Alternatively, weakness in the quad muscles can lead to increased loading force going through the knee, another driver of irritation in this region. This ratio changes depending on the task at hand and is much less critical in easier-paced runs compared to higher-intensity intervals. Further down the chain, increased pronation in the ankle can contribute to medial loading on the knee due to too much rotation of the tibia. On the other hand, tightness in the calves or ankle can restrict the small amount of rotation that is necessary at the tibiofemoral joint, leading to increased torque at the knee as the femur continues to rotate but the knee gets "stuck." As you can see, there are many non-knee factors that can contribute to pain in the knee.

To make matters more complicated, multiple areas in the knee are prone to irritation. For instance, iliotibial band (IT band) injury presents as knee pain and is so common that we have dedicated a whole chapter (chapter 14) to helping you sort through it. For pain behind the knee (insertional hamstrings), you can find answers in our chapter on hamstrings (chapter 13). This chapter focuses primarily on injuries due to the mechanics of the knee, covering runner's knee (patellofemoral pain syndrome), patellar and quadriceps tendinitis, and meniscal injury.

Patellofemoral Pain Syndrome (PFPS)

Patellofemoral pain syndrome, PFPS, also known as runner's knee, is somewhat of a catchall term. It loosely refers to inflammation of the kneecap, or patella, and its surrounding structures (cartilage, tendons, ligaments, retinaculum, and fat pad). Classic symptoms of PFPS include pain around the knee or under the patella during and after running, especially going up and down stairs, and increased pain after sitting at your desk or on your couch for a few hours.

Diagnosis

PFPS is often associated with increased "crunchiness," or what a doctor may call *crepitus*, around the knee joint. It may be accompanied by swelling around the knee, with pain usually isolated to the area around the kneecap or on the inside of the knee.

One reason your knee might be crunchy is tightness in the structures around the knee (quad muscles, IT band, hamstring muscles) increasing compression of the patellar tendon as it glides across the knee joint during activity. There can also be restrictions in the knee retinaculum—the dense, connective tissue that surrounds the knee joint. If the problem stems specifically from the cartilage underneath your kneecap, the diagnosis may be *chondromalacia patellae*, meaning that the cartilage has softened or begun to deteriorate. In this instance, instead of gliding smoothly, there is more friction as the knee bends back and forth. You might feel an uncomfortable cracking in the knee when bending it back and forth, standing up after sitting for a while, or walking up and down stairs.

If you think that you may have PFPS caused by running, the next step is to identify any mechanical problems that may be at the root of the injury. Some research suggests that the drivers are a little different between women and men, mainly due to women typically having a wider-set pelvis than men, causing a greater loading angle, termed *Q angle*, at the knee joint on landing (Noehren et al. 2021; Willy et al. 2012). This puts more stress on the inside of the knee. People who demonstrate increased femoral internal rotation and adduction (figure 7.3*a*) when they land (knee valgus) and increased hip drop (figure 7.3*b*) have increased risk of developing PFPS compared to runners who are able to maintain proper form (figure 7.3*c*).

No matter your gender, having a weak core and hip muscles can contribute to PFPS. Your gluteus maximus muscle works as a powerful hip external rotator and abductor, countering the internal rotation and adduction forces

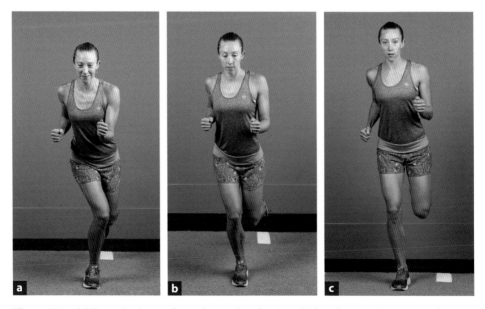

Figure 7.3   *(a)* Excessive internal rotation and adduction, *(b)* hip drop, and *(c)* proper form on landing.

of landing. Your core and other hip muscles (gluteus medius, gluteus mini-mis, and adductors) help to hold your hips level when you land. Weakness in your core and hip muscles is connected with hip drop and increased valgus on landing, both of which can lead to PFPS.

Finally, increased pronation in the foot can also play a role in PFPS, but uncontrolled pronation is more likely a result of weakness in the hips, which may be causing the knee pain. Overstriding is linked with increased force through the knee and can also contribute to PFPS.

Treatment

As with most running injuries, the first thing to assess is your training. Did you ramp up mileage too fast without allowing for the adequate tissue adaptations? This, in combination with the risk factors listed earlier, is a surefire way to instigate knee pain.

After reducing the load on your body from overly aggressive training, the next step is to assess and treat tightness that might be at the root of your pain. If tension in the structures around your knee is the driving cause of your PFPS, strategies to loosen up these areas are critical to reducing the load being placed on the kneecap. Both deep tissue massage and cupping, or myofascial compression and decompression, can be helpful in adjunct with other treatment methods for decreasing stress on the knee.

Those of us who sit at desks all day are at considerably greater risk of developing tightness that can lead to PFPS. Here are a few tips to keep moving during the day to help prevent and recover from PFPS:

- Keep your knees moving back and forth, bending all the way and straightening to help improve blood flow and circulation. Try these movements with the ankle twisted inward and outward to increase tibial internal and external rotation.
- Stand, walk around, and perform some deep squats and hip stretches throughout the day to keep your hip joints moving and to decrease tension in the quads and hip flexors.
- If you are rehabilitating PFPS, sit with the injured leg propped up straight instead of bent beneath you. This position limits the amount of fluid that can enter the knee, which will decrease your pain with movements (although it can contribute to stiffness, so make sure to keep moving).

At home, foam rolling the quads and hamstrings is an effective way to increase tissue mobility, thus reducing the force and compression that they transmit into the patellofemoral joint. We recommend foam rolling both before and after running to help improve tissue extensibility.

Stretching the quadriceps muscles and hip flexors is also critical to keep your pelvis moving well, and adequate mobility at the hip and ankle joints is equally critical. We break these down in more detail in the chapters on the ankle and the hip. See chapter 6 for the 3D calf stretch and ankle pronation and supination, and see chapter 8 for more detailed instructions on performing the hip floss and 3D pivots, our favorite exercises for hip mobility.

The 3D kneeling hip flexor stretch is absolutely one of the best ways to stretch your quads and mobilize your pelvis. While you are working on tight areas contributing to your PFPS, strengthening the glutes and muscles around the knee will help to decrease the load on the knee. The exercises after the 3D kneeling hip flexor stretch will accomplish that.

3D Kneeling Hip Flexor Stretch

Start by kneeling on a pillow or soft surface. One leg will be in front of you flat footed with knee bent, while you are kneeling on the other leg. Make sure you emphasize tucking your pelvis slightly and engaging your core; if you are overarching your lower back, the stretch will be much less productive (figure 7.4*a*). Begin shifting your hips forward and backward. Then place a hand on your hip bone and reach the opposite arm up, to drive your pelvis laterally (you are reaching the arm up that is on the same side as the kneeling leg up and overhead, toward the other side). You should feel an increased stretch through your psoas and side. Switch arms—now you'll drive the other way, so the arm on the opposite side of the kneeling leg is reaching up and overhead (figure 7.4*b*). This time, you should feel an increased stretch in the inside of your leg. Finally, rotate your pelvis inward and outward. This dynamic stretch helps to mobilize both the quadriceps and the pelvis in all three planes of motion, which helps take pressure off your knee. Switch sides and repeat on the other hip.

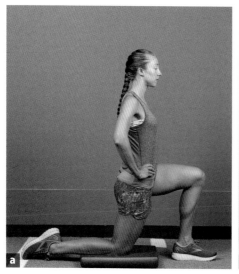 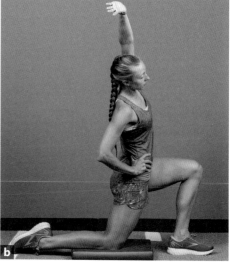

Figure 7.4 3D kneeling hip flexor stretch: *(a)* start position; *(b)* lateral stretch with arm up.

3D kneeling hip flexor stretch learned from Gray Institute®, GrayInstitute.com.

Long Arc Quad

This exercise is very simple and easy to do at your desk and throughout the day while seated in a chair. Straighten your knee and then slowly bend your knee, lowering your foot to the ground (figure 7.5*a* and figure 7.5*b*), working on eccentric control. If you feel any discomfort, stop at that point in the movement; you want to stay in the pain-free range. We recommend adding an ankle weight, as this exercise will begin to feel pretty easy very quickly. You can also replicate this exercise at the gym with the leg extension machine on the lightest setting. Perform it on the leg extension machine with one leg only.

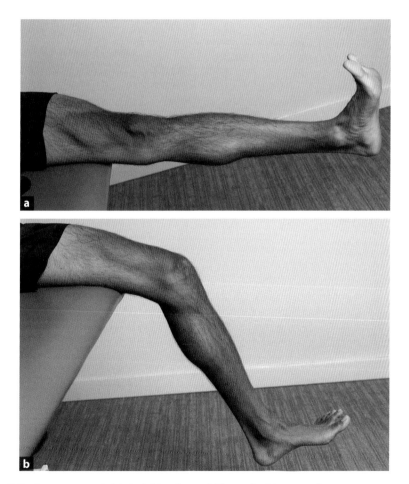

Figure 7.5   Long arc quad: *(a)* straighten knee; *(b)* lower foot to ground.

Single-Leg Split Squat
(Bulgarian Split Squat)

Stand on one foot with the other foot elevated on a bench or box behind you that is approximately knee height or slightly lower. Keeping your weight on your front heel, sit back into your hips. Your front knee should bend second to your hips flexing, making sure you aren't feeling any pressure in the front of your knee (figure 7.6). Focus on slowly controlling the downward movement with your front quad muscles. Push up through your heel, using your glutes and hamstrings to drive up.

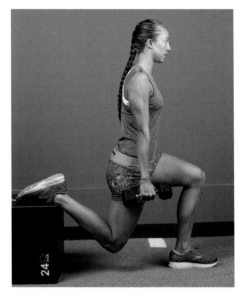

Figure 7.6   Single-leg split squat.

Adductor Strengthening

The adductors are often overlooked, but this muscle group helps stabilize the pelvis when we land and helps us smoothly transition from one leg to another. Weakness or dysfunction in the adductors can be a driving factor behind both knee and hip pain. Increased femoral external rotation can keep adductors in an overlengthened position, which prevents the adductors from helping to stabilize the leg and pelvis when a runner lands. It can also be a reason for medial knee pain or hip dysfunction.

When doing any type of lunging exercise, focus on keeping the knee straight, so it stays over your toes rather than veering left or right. An easy way to increase adductor engagement in a variety of exercises is simply to pay attention to which way your leg is tracking—is it able to stay straight and aligned with your pelvis and your foot? To increase adductor engagement, loop a resistance band laterally around a stable object such as a pole and then around the working thigh (so you have an outward force) while performing lunges and squats; this forces the adductor to work harder to help keep the leg stable.

Lateral Toe Taps

With a resistance band around both knees (above the knees to start; if this gets easier, you can move to below the knees), sink back so you are sitting into your glutes. Make sure your knees are not extending past your toes and you don't feel any pressure in your knees (you can hold onto a chair or counter if needed to maintain balance). Shift all your weight into one leg and keep your weight rooted through your heel. The stance leg should not move. With your other leg, reach out diagonally to the side and slightly backward and tap your foot lightly, as if you were tapping eggshells (figure 7.7). Repeat 10 times on each side as a warm-up, or do three sets of 10 if you're doing lateral taps as part of a strength routine.

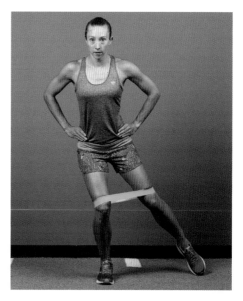

Figure 7.7 Lateral toe taps.

Monster Walks

With a looped resistance band around your knees, or around your ankles for more of a challenge, sink back into your glutes, keeping your weight posteriorly loaded (as opposed to through your knees and quads). Staying as low and steady as you can, take a controlled step to the side (figure 7.8). Think about pushing off with the side glute on your trailing leg. Take 10 to 15 steps in one direction (left or right), then reverse direction and take 10 to 15 steps back.

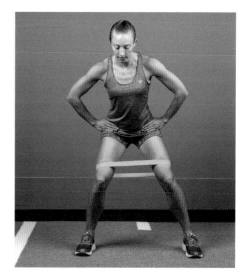

Figure 7.8 Monster walks.

Case Study: Brianna

Brianna reports to her physical therapist that she recently increased her running and is having a lot of pain on the insides of her knees. She reports that the pain feels like it's behind the kneecap.

Observation: In conjunction with her presenting pain and testing positive for weakness in her quads, glutes, and transverse abdominis, Brianna's running form demonstrates increased dynamic valgus on loading, with excessive hip adduction and internal rotation, paired with compensatory external rotation of her lower leg to help her push off. Brianna has not done much strength training.

Diagnosis: Patellofemoral pain syndrome (chondromalacia patellae).

Treatment: Treatment begins with manual therapy, including soft tissue work around the knees to improve blood flow and tissue mobility of the knee retinaculum, the connective tissue or fascia that surrounds the knee joint. Brianna also responds well to athletic taping, a technique designed to improve circulation and relative movement between the layers of the knee retinaculum, as well as to increase the proprioceptive sense of stability. A quad, glute, and hamstring strengthening program helps Brianna better stabilize her pelvis in landing, and she revises her training program to include a gradual increase in mileage while she works on improving her running form with regular drills.

Finally, alongside enhanced strength training, using real-time cueing and biofeedback to improve form can help treat and prevent PFPS (Willy, Scholz, and Davis 2012). While this can't be taught in a book, a few sessions with a physical therapist, coach, or other movement professional can help you to integrate needed changes into your stride.

Patellar and Quadriceps Tendinitis and Tendinosis

Unlike PFPS, patellar and quadriceps tendinitis and tendinosis, also known as jumper's knee, tend to be more localized to the specific structure that is inflamed. The easiest way that this type of injury can be distinguished from PFPS is that the region of pain is definable and the area of the patellar–quadriceps tendon is painful to touch. You might notice stiffness in the morning that gets better with activity or feel the most pain at the beginning of a run, but then the pain will ease, only to return after your run. Unlike PFPS, you are unlikely to have pain that worsens with rest.

Patellar tendinitis is inflammation of the patellar tendon, the tendon directly below the kneecap that connects the patella to the tibia. The patellar tendon helps to transfer the force of the powerful quadriceps muscles to the lower leg to effectively and efficiently straighten the knee. In running, the patellar tendon also plays a huge role in shock absorption: As the knee bends to absorb the force of the leg hitting the ground, the patellar tendon transfers the load from the quads through the lower leg.

The quadriceps tendon is positioned above the kneecap and connects the quadriceps muscles to the bone. Like any tendon in your body, it is designed for efficient transfer of load and is a thick, dense structure of connective tissue. Unlike the actual muscle belly of the quadriceps, if the quadriceps tendon becomes inflamed due to excessive overload, it can take a long time to fully heal. Therefore, identifying the injury correctly is necessary so that proper treatment protocol and activity modification can be undertaken as early as possible.

While patellar tendinitis is more common in runners than quadriceps tendinitis, distinguishing which of the two structures is inflamed can help to streamline the recovery process, because focus can be put on the area of irritation. Risk factors for developing patellar and quadriceps tendinitis include weakness or disuse in your quads, calves, or glute muscles. Remember, weakness can be relative. Even with adequate strength training, you need to learn to engage these muscles when you run. Weakness in these muscle groups can cause increased reliance on tendons for running economy. Additionally, it can cause increased localized strain on the tendon due to unequal force distribution (Van Gent et al. 2007).

Tightness and overuse in the hip flexors and quadriceps muscles can also drive tendinitis in this part of the body. Similar to Achilles tendinitis, inflammation and pain can result if the peritenon, the connective tissue that surrounds the patellar or quadriceps tendon, gets restricted and movement is not fluid. A driving factor in this type of restriction is tightness and stiffness in the quad muscles.

Treatment

As discussed in chapter 6, tendinitis—in this case, in the quadriceps and patellar tendon—can progress to tendinosis after four to six weeks. The stage of the injury affects the way we treat it.

If you notice tendinitis during its initial onset, we recommend pausing your running training. Light cross-training on the bike or in the pool is okay, and you'll want to start performing pain-free isometric strengthening (i.e., static contraction of the muscles, such as the wall sit exercise on page 71). The goal is to prevent the injury from worsening and, consequently, requiring more rehab. If the injury has persisted for more than six weeks and turned to tendinosis, rehab can be a little more aggressive. Pushing through some minor discomfort when running is permissible. This doesn't mean you should go out and hammer workouts, but maintaining easy mileage while also working on rehabbing your knee is generally okay, depending on how severe the tendinosis is. If you aren't sure where your injury falls within this range, we recommend consulting with a health care professional.

Several types of exercises are effective for tendon healing as part of a rehab and strength program for patellar and quadriceps tendon injury. It's important that the tendon receives adequate stress to promote healing, but not so much that it's being overloaded and reaggravated. Eccentric strengthening is considered the gold standard for tendinopathy treatment. Both heavy slow resistance training (such as one-repetition maximum (1RM); Rio et al. 2016) and isometric contractions (Rio et al. 2015) have been shown to reduce pain, improve collagen turnover, increase strength, and improve function in patellar tendinopathies. New research supports the benefits of increased loading and strength training (Rio et al. 2015, 2016). We recommend starting with isometric resistance training (resisted static contraction) and progressing to eccentric loading (declined squat, single leg squat) as well as heavy, slow resistance training (e.g., 1RM of a split squat).

Progressive Loading Program

Here we outline a progressive loading exercise program for tendinopathy of the knee. We can't emphasize enough how important it is to also consult with your doctor or physical therapist to make sure this is appropriate for you.

A general rule to follow as you progress through this (or another) rehab program: If your pain levels are less than 3 out of 10 and are not increasing with activity, it's okay to push through. If you aren't sure, once again, check in with your doctor.

TABLE 7.1   Progressive Loading Program for Patellar and Quadriceps Tendinitis and Tendinosis

Weeks	Focus	Exercises
1-2	Blood flow Pain relief	Long arc quad Wall sit
3-4	Progressive loading Weight-bearing control	Eccentric squat on an incline board Double-leg squat, progressing weight Single-leg squat, progressing weight
5-6	Increasing weight as tolerated	-
7-8	Plyometric control Multidirectional control Suspected and unsuspected movement changes	Plyometric drills, double and single leg Box jumps, double and single leg Multidirectional hops, double and single leg

Weeks 1-2

The goal of this phase of rehab is to encourage blood flow to the tendon and reduce pain. It is also helpful to incorporate general glute, hip, and core strengthening at this phase of rehab, which will indirectly help to take pressure off the knee without exacerbating symptoms. The long arc quad exercise is described earlier in this chapter (see figure 7.5).

Wall Sit

Start with two or three 40-second wall sits. With your back against the wall, engage your abs and slowly slide your back down until your thighs are parallel to the ground, positioning your knees over your ankles, not your toes. Take approximately one minute of rest between each wall sit to recover. You can add manual resistance to create isometric abduction and adduction contractions, further activating and engaging the supporting muscles around the knee. Add manual resistance to leg abduction and adduction by pushing your hand against your leg and your leg back against your hand with equal pressure so your leg doesn't actually move. Put your hand on the outside of your leg and push for leg abduction (10 seconds; figure 7.9a). Put your hand on the inside of your leg and push for leg adduction (10 seconds; figure 7.9b).

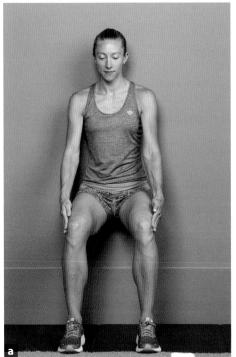 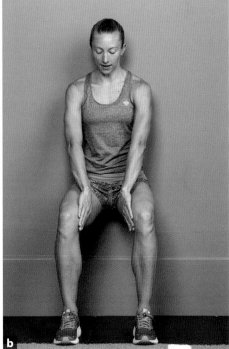

Figure 7.9   Wall sit: *(a)* abduction; *(b)* adduction.

Weeks 3-4

This phase of rehab is focused on progressive loading in a weight-bearing position, starting with two legs and progressing to one leg and increasing the weight. Focus on proper form, load distribution, and engaging your quads on the descent while using your posterior chain (glutes and hamstrings) to push back up.

Eccentric Squat on an Incline Board

These are very slow squats performed with your ankles raised on an incline board or very low step (figure 7.10). Focus on slowing your squat so the eccentric contractions of your leg muscles are smooth and controlled. The incline board puts your ankles in a plantar flexed position, which functionally lessens the use of the calf muscles in your squat. Because of this, your quads and hamstrings will need to work harder. Perform three sets of 15 squats twice a day.

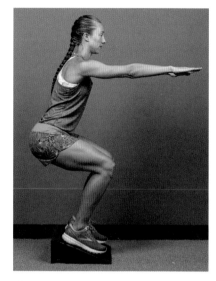

Figure 7.10 Eccentric squat on an incline board.

Double-Leg Squat

On level ground, begin by squatting with both feet flat on the floor (figure 7.11). We suggest doing this in front of a mirror, to make sure you are evenly distributing your load and are not shifting more weight onto the uninjured side. If you are able to perform three sets of 10 squats pain-free with no compensation, slowly add weight by holding two lightweight dumbbells, and see what effort it takes to perform 10. If the effort is minimal, add another pound. Continue this until you can perform 10 squats with dumbbells at a moderate effort level.

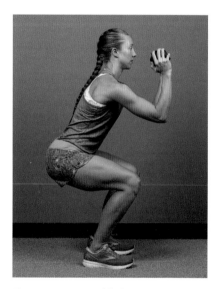

Figure 7.11 Double-leg squat.

Single-Leg Squat

Once your double-leg squat is pain-free and you are plateauing on effort level, add single-leg squats. (You will continue with the double-leg squat; you're merely adding single-leg squats to the repertoire.) For this exercise, all of your weight should be on one leg, and your floating leg should reach behind you, toes tapping the ground very lightly, like a kickstand (figure 7.12). Begin just as you did for double-leg squats; perform 10 without any weight first to focus on form and control. Switch legs after 10 repetitions. Add modest weight and progress until you can perform 10 repetitions with moderate effort and minimal to no knee pain. Progress to 70 to 85 percent of 1 rep max as tolerated.

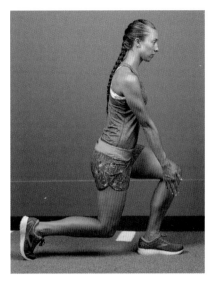

Figure 7.12 Single-leg squat.

Weeks 5-6

Continue with previous exercises and increase weight.

Weeks 7-8

The six-week mark is usually the earliest point at which a patient will be cleared to begin engaging in plyometric training; week seven is a surer bet for more conservative professionals and patients. This final stage of rehabilitation for runners is the most task-specific. By increasing tolerance to higher-level plyometric training, we are increasing the buffer zone in which our tendons can respond to advanced loading and power moves. Because most runners engage in relatively minor plyometric movements, incorporating advanced training designed to increase power is immensely beneficial in increasing resilience through the tissue. You can handle more miles and more intense training with less fatigue, have less form breakdown, and risk injury less.

Box Jumps

Begin by facing a sturdy box or step about six inches off the floor. Raise your arms toward the ceiling, bring them down as you sit back into your hips, and as you jump, propel your arms with your momentum. Lift your knees, and try to land as softly as possible (figure 7.13). Step down, and repeat 10 times. To progress this exercise, raise the height of the box. You can also jump and land on one leg at a time.

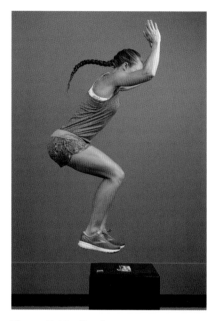

Figure 7.13   Box jumps.

Multidirectional Hops

Starting on two feet, jump forward and backward for 30 seconds (figure 7.14). Then jump side to side (left and right) for 30 seconds. Finally, twist your body to jump rotationally left and right for 30 seconds. As you get stronger, you should be able to hop farther. To progress this exercise, perform the hops on one foot instead of two.

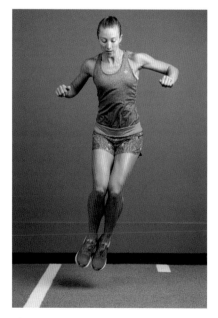

Figure 7.14   Multidirectional hops.

Similarly to treatment for PFPS, we also recommend foam rolling your quads and hamstrings and stretching your hips to help to off-load the tension around your knee. See the section on foam rolling in chapter 8 for further details.

Working on form is especially important for healing and preventing this injury from recurring. New research suggests that muscle strengthening alone is not enough to "cure" tendinitis. Instead, a combination of muscle strengthening and activation *and* proper movement retraining is critical for return to sport (Rio et al. 2016). Increasing your running cadence and incorporating running form drills (which you can read about in chapter 16) make a great starting place.

Case Study: Mark

Mark reports that he recently started a new training program that upped his running mileage and intensity. After a tough hill workout last week, he reports that he felt a sudden onset of pain in both knees. He expresses confusion, saying "I don't understand—my body should be able to handle it because I lift weights two or three times every week!"

Observation: Mark presents with very strong quads but very poor hip extension. When squatting, Mark has difficulty engaging his glutes and hamstrings and shifting weight into the backs of his legs. Mark's calves are more defined and muscular than muscles up the chain. He does not engage his core well with dynamic movements. Mark exhibits cross-chain syndrome (figure 7.15). In cross-chain syndrome, the quads become very tight, pulling the pelvis into an anterior pelvic tilt, causing the core to over-lengthen.

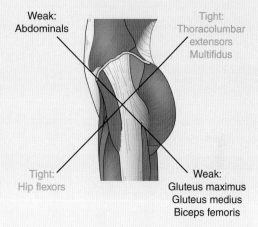

Figure 7.15 Cross-chain syndrome.

The low back compensates for the weak core by tightening and overworking. This prevents the glutes from being able to extend and help the posterior chain, often causing increased tightness in the calves. The calves, quads, and low back are tight and overworked and the glutes, core, and hamstrings are weak and underworked.

Diagnosis: Patellar tendinitis.

Treatment: Mark reduces his training volume and begins a home regimen of foam rolling and stretching his quad muscles before and after all runs. By improving his hip mobility and working on glute strengthening, he is better able to use his glutes when he runs, which leads to decreased overstriding and force through his knees when he lands. He also incorporates a wall sit into his prerun warm-up routine; this stabilizes his joints and increases muscle recruitment of the fibers surrounding his knee. Separately, he begins an eccentric strength training program and works with a coach to correct his overstriding. He also consults the coach about better balancing his strength training with his running program to allow for proper recovery.

Meniscus

Meniscal injury in runners can be divided into two types: a *traumatic* tear that happens because of a misstep such as tripping off a curb, over a dog, or down a rocky trail, or a *degenerative* injury that happens gradually over time due to wear and tear of the joint. Pain in the meniscus (figure 7.16) will feel deeper than PFPS or tendinitis. You may have some tenderness right at the joint line, and the area will feel especially irritated with twisting or rotational movements or deep bending of the knee. In severe cases of a meniscus tear, surgery may be necessary, but proper treatment can often resolve symptoms without resorting to surgery. Plus, because running typically does not involve much rotational movement, you can often continue to run while you are treating this injury, with only a few modifications.

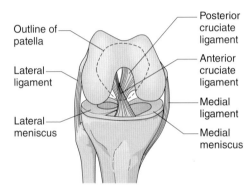

Figure 7.16   Meniscus.

Onset

A traumatic meniscal injury causes a sharp pain in the knee, perhaps with an associated popping or clicking sound when walking. Somewhat counter-intuitively, a person with a traumatic meniscal injury may find that running is one of the few things they can do without pain. This is because running typically doesn't require the knee to react to outside rotational forces. However, beware of a stray soccer ball flying across the track, and don't plan on joining your friends on a trail run, because any exaggerated or unexpected movement could aggravate the injury.

Alternatively, a degenerative meniscal injury is likely due to abnormal rotation patterns in the tibia or femur. This is more commonly caused by trail running or other repetitive running on uneven surfaces. As discussed at the beginning of the chapter, if rotation is off-track at the ankle or the hip, the knee gets stuck in the middle trying to compensate and therefore undergoes more motion than it can handle. In this case, the meniscus bears the brunt of the excessive and uneven load distribution that's traveling through the knee.

Treatment

If you suspect that your knee pain may be stemming from the meniscus, we first recommend running only on smooth, flat, soft surfaces, like a bike path or running track. (The straighter the path, the better.) Because the meniscus works as a sort of cushion or shock absorber for the knee, soft surfaces can help reduce load and impact being managed by the meniscus. Avoid any type of surface or route that has bumps, potholes, or children riding bicycles to ensure that you don't need to suddenly move laterally or twist, which can aggravate the meniscus.

Because of the structure of the meniscus, the area doesn't get a lot of fresh blood, so its capacity for full healing is limited. This sounds scary, but what it means is that rehab must focus on improving joint mechanics to reduce irritation to the knee. Therefore, we strongly advise an evaluation by a movement professional in order to determine if you have excessive femoral internal rotation driven by weak glutes, increased tibial external rotation driven by tight calves, or ankle stiffness—all of which can be hard to tease out on your own. In the meantime, foam rolling your quads, strengthening your hip external rotators, doing exercises that control femoral internal rotation, rolling and loosening up the calves, and working on ankle pronation and supination can be helpful and safe additions to your routine. (See chapter 6 for further instruction on ankle pronation and supination.)

Case Study: Jade

Jade was running in her neighborhood when a dog cut across her path and she fell. Since then, she reports that her knee just hasn't felt right. She can get through most of her runs without much pain, but then it will hurt sporadically, like when she pivots to avoid a car, and sometimes when stepping on or off a curb.

Observation: Jade demonstrates good tolerance to all sagittal plane (forward and backward) movements but is unable to disassociate her pelvis from her femur with any movements. She can run pain-free but has difficulty turning or negotiating any obstacle.

Diagnosis: Meniscal injury (confirmed with MRI).

Treatment: Jade's treatment program involves manual therapy and soft tissue manipulation to the fascia around her knee and joint line. She also performs a series of mobility exercises (pivots, hip floss, three-way lunges) focused on increasing her pelvic range of motion and ability to move her pelvis separately from her hip and strengthening her hip muscles, quads, hamstrings, and adductors. This allows Jade to move better without torquing her knee.

Case Study: Jamie

Jamie was on a 10-mile trail run (a type of run she doesn't normally do) when she suddenly felt a snap in her knee. Jamie also reports that she was in her highest mileage week of training in her marathon buildup and had done a tough workout the day before. She was able to finish the run but is having some swelling in her knee. She is also feeling pain and a clicking sensation when she walks.

Observation: This case highlights how overtraining can also lead to meniscal injury. Jamie's muscles were too fatigued to adequately support her, mechanically, when running, and she experienced excessive rotational forces in her knee on the trail, which stressed the meniscus past its load capacity.

Diagnosis: Meniscal tear.

Treatment: Jamie ended up having surgery to remove the torn part of her meniscus because she continued to experience her knee "locking up on her" and severe pain in her day-to-day activities. Following surgery, her rehab program included strengthening exercises for the hips and muscles around the knee, mobility work focused on improving rotation at the hip and the ankle, form adjustments, and a training plan that allowed for adequate recovery between runs.

Proactively Preventing Knee Injury

As with many other injuries, the single easiest controllable factor for preventing knee injury is proper training. Make sure you aren't ramping up your distance or intensity too quickly. The next easiest factor to control is running surface. Try your best to run on grass or dirt whenever possible. Number three is cadence. Shorter, quicker steps can reduce overstriding and decrease the amount of impact that is going through your leg—and therefore knee—with each step. Increasing cadence to closer to 180 steps per minute has been linked to decreasing overuse injuries and knee pain in runners.

The fourth is mobility. Tightness in the quads, hip flexors, and calves is a common theme in many knee injuries. This tightness restricts proper joint kinematics, limiting hip extension and tibial rotation, which reduce force and load at the knee in running. The ankle also factors in, because restrictions through the lower leg can translate to either increased or decreased rotation at the knee.

Finally, the fifth element we recommend working on is weakness. Core weakness can lead to overrecruitment of hip flexors and quadriceps muscles for stability. Overuse of the quads can be a driver behind knee pain, which can result from a compensation due to weak core muscles. Weakness in the quad muscles can also lead to increased force through the knee, because of the quads' role in shock absorption. Weakness in your glute muscles can lead to increased knee valgus, compression through the patella, and a lack of ability to resist rotational forces. This means you might not respond as well to a misstep, and you aren't as good at stabilizing your body in landing.

Sometimes, weak glutes can stem from tightness in your quads and hip flexors; because of restrictions in the front of the hip, you aren't able to extend your hip and fully access your glutes, which is why we advise addressing mobility before looking at strength.

Conclusion

This final list of five proactive measures is great for preventing knee injuries, but that doesn't mean knee injuries won't happen. If you do feel pain around your knee, we recommend getting an evaluation by a movement professional who specializes in running injuries. Often non-sport-specific medical professionals will hear that you have knee pain and when you tell them you run, they'll immediately assume there is structural damage to the knee. However, as you learned in this chapter, the problem may not stem from the knee itself but from other causal factors creating irritation in or around the knee. A movement professional will help determine if increased femoral internal rotation or decreased tibial external rotation is at the root of your knee pain issues.

CHAPTER 8

Hips

While legs and feet often get the spotlight when it comes to running, body parts up the chain are also very involved. Hips, for instance, are key. Hip injury in runners can come in a variety of shapes and sizes. In this chapter we outline and connect the driving factors of hip injury, discuss the most common hip injuries that plague runners, and provide you with tips for preventing injury.

How Hip Injuries Arise

Although running is primarily a forward movement, there are components of gait that include side to side and rotational movements that originate from your hip. The catch is that many of us spend a large portion of our day sitting. Over time, this can severely impact the accessible range of motion in the hip. Compensatory patterns emerge, and these patterns can be factors behind hip injury.

A common reason this happens is an imbalance that you are probably familiar with by this point—increased tightness and restrictions in the front of the hip and weakness in the muscle groups that stabilize the hips, including the glutes and core.

There are significant differences between the hips of women and men. Men typically have a narrower pelvis, which adds more stability to the region and decreases excessive torquing forces. Women have a wider pelvis that eases delivery in childbirth. Because of a wider pelvis, however, the amount of force that transmits through a woman's hip during running is greater, increasing the likelihood of hip and knee injury. Furthermore, hormones specific to pregnancy and breastfeeding increase the amount of laxity or looseness and stretchiness in the ligaments that support the hip. This can make people who have been pregnant more prone to injury in this region. Strengthening the abs and muscles surrounding the pelvis can therefore play a critical role in reducing risk of injury to the hips, especially during the prenatal and postpartum period.

Anatomy of the Hip Joint

The hip is one of the most complex joints in the body; it's designed to do a lot. Primarily, the hip is designed to move. The joint is shaped like a ball-

and-socket, with ample degrees of mobility in all three planes of motion (figure 8.1). It is crucial that the femur (thigh bone) can move forward and back, side to side, and rotationally on the pelvis (hip bone). Equally imperative is the ability of the pelvis to move forward and back, side to side, and rotationally on the femur.

Limitations in hip mobility can lead to many unhealthy compensatory strategies. A stiff hip can make it tough to access the range of motion necessary to recruit the muscles that propel the leg forward (e.g., weak glutes that just don't seem to get stronger, no matter how many bridges you do). Stiff hips can also lead to compensatory excessive movement in the joints above and below the hips, specifically the low back and knees, two regions of the body that are designed for stability, not mobility. The hip is designed to rotate to a much greater extent than the knees and the low back. This puts us in a chicken-or-egg scenario: Does tightness in the hips lead to weak muscles and bad compensations, or do weak muscles keep us from moving our hips properly, contributing to hip tightness?

The hips also need to have a strong core with which to work. A strong, stable core is necessary to support the large amount of motion needed at the hip and to allow this critical joint to work properly. Weakness in the core can also play a role in increased stiffness at the hip. The body is looking for stability from somewhere, and if it isn't able to adequately stabilize in the abdomen, the hip flexors take over. Not only can this lead to hip issues, it can also be a player in gastrointestinal distress, pelvic floor dysfunction, and a whole host of other problems!

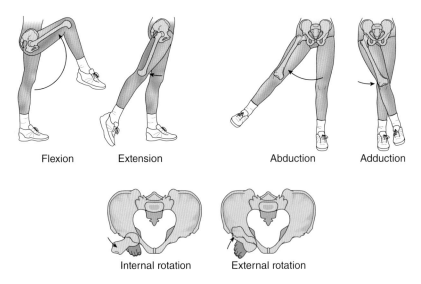

Flexion   Extension   Abduction   Adduction

Internal rotation   External rotation

Figure 8.1   Triplanar hip movement.

How the Hip Works in Running

The hip is the power driver for runners. It functions like a slingshot, stretching on impact to allow for a strong elastic recoil on push-off that propels the runner forward. While you might be able to get away with tight hips when running slower paces, if you ever try to attempt something more up-tempo, hip mobility is critical. The three-dimensional motion of the hip allows runners to glide and flow forward properly, engaging the glutes. The hip assists in sharing the workload of the calves, hamstrings, and low back, so that no muscle group is overworked.

When a runner lands, the hip joint moves into flexion, adduction, and internal rotation as the head of the femur glides and spins backward in the socket (figure 8.2). This mechanism transfers the ground reaction force into the glute muscle, and the glute muscle uses this force to propel the runner forward. Think of this like a slingshot or rubber band: On landing, the rubber band (glute) stretches and then recoils like a spring or elastic. Tightness in the hips and pelvis can limit this loading mechanism. When this happens, compensation is quick to occur. Lack of rotation can lead to overworking of the quads and hip flexors. If we aren't getting this springy recoil mechanism from the pelvis, we are more likely to become overly dependent on using our quads and hip flexors to drive us forward. This can pull the pelvis forward into a faulty alignment, leading to hip impingement, tendinitis, or other overuse injuries in the front of the hip. Limitations in side-to-side movement can lead to iliotibial (IT) band injury or greater trochanteric bursitis.

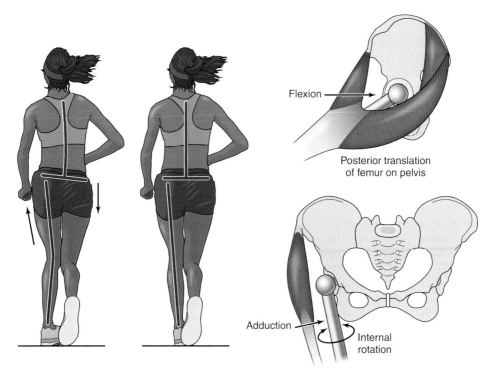

Figure 8.2 Loading mechanism of the hip.

Understanding Hip Injury

The most common injuries that plague the hip are interconnected, stemming from several principles. We will briefly overview hip pathology, but what you should understand from this chapter is that maintaining hip health is extremely important, especially given the world of cars and computers that we live in. By learning how to properly care for your hip joint, many common hip injuries can be avoided.

Labral Pathology

The labrum of your hip is the tissue that lines the inside of your hip joint socket. It functions as a cushion for the joint, allows the head of the femur to glide smoothly in all directions, and also helps to stabilize the joint. A labrum injury involves a tearing, fraying, or inflammation that can cause pain that radiates out into the hip region. If you have been diagnosed with a labral tear, your doctor may have mentioned surgery. Give treatment and rehab a shot first. Labral injuries can often be treated successfully by a physical therapist.

Restrictions in the hip joint that prevent the femoral head from gliding smoothly in the socket can lead to a "snagging," which can irritate and injure the labrum. If the labrum is inflamed, look at overall strength, imbalance, and restrictions. Often, labral injuries are paired with a tightness in the hip flexors that limits the posterior glide and rotation of the femoral head into the socket. This leads to a less than optimal distribution of forces through the joint with landing.

Groin Injury

Groin injuries can be some of the trickiest for runners to deal with, and there are many different kinds. A runner suffering groin pain might be diagnosed with athletic pubalgia, osteitis pubis, sports hernia, or insertional adductor tendinitis, among others.

Groin injuries often stem from common root causes. If your pelvis is rotated too far forward (anterior pelvic tilt) or you have externally rotated femurs, this can cause muscles that attach to the pelvis to function in a mechanically disadvantageous position. Specifically, the rectus abdominis (your six pack muscle) becomes overlengthened, which places excessive strain on the pubic symphysis (Moran and Rogowski 2020). In femoral external rotation, the adductors begin to function like your quadriceps muscle and also become overworked and tight. Alternatively, these muscles may be weak and unable to adequately stabilize the pelvis. Over time, this can lead to inflammation of the pubic symphysis, groin, and ligaments that stabilize the pelvis. Therefore, proper alignment and the ability to function in a neutral position are critical.

Hip Impingement

Hip impingement is caused when there is too much friction in the hip joint, specifically between the hip socket of the pelvis and the thigh bone (femur). In simpler terms, it's a pinching or jamming of the hip joint. Hip impingement is often due to excessive bony overgrowth of the pelvis or femur and is common in younger athletes. However, hip impingement can also be functional, meaning that due to pelvic malalignment, tight muscles, or restrictions in the joint, the hip is compressed and becomes jammed. Hip impingement can be a reason for groin injury, tendinitis, or hip labral tears.

Hip Tendinitis

Tendinitis is often the result of muscle imbalance. Either a muscle is working too hard to make up for another muscle that isn't pulling its weight, or a muscle is weak and becomes overloaded, leading to inflammation of the tendon. In the hip, if a muscle is functioning in a disadvantageous position, it's also more prone to tendon inflammation, or tendinitis.

Hip Bursitis

Hip bursitis can appear on the side of the hip, in the greater trochanteric bursa, or, less commonly, in the front of the hip, the iliopsoas bursa. Bursitis has a similar etiology to tendinitis, although occasionally it can be caused by a direct trauma or fall, so be careful if you are running in icy conditions or on an uneven surface. The greater trochanteric bursa sits on the side of the hip, and its primary job is to provide lubrication to the hip joint so that the tendons can move with less friction. When overloaded, the bursa can become inflamed and cause pain, usually stemming from a combination of overtraining and faulty mechanics. As is the common theme of this chapter, weak glutes or poor hip mobility can cause too much lateral loading when the foot hits the ground, and, similar to the etiology of IT band syndrome (see chapter 14), the bursa can become irritated.

Hidden Pelvic or Femoral Neck Stress Fracture

A stress fracture of the pelvic bone or femoral neck (the part of the femur that attaches to the pelvis) is often sneakily hidden at the hip joint. Because of the interconnectedness of the hip, stress fractures usually present as something else and go undiagnosed. This puts the runner at high risk of a full fracture. A fractured pelvis or femoral neck is very serious; in fact, it is the most serious of all stress fractures. A runner with this injury risks an actual collapse of the hip, which requires surgery to place metal hardware in the hip to stabilize it. Recovery from this injury can take more than a year.

The classic signs of a pelvic stress fracture are limping when walking, consistent pain with impact (landing during walking or running), and difficulty in alleviating the pain with other treatments. Pain when shifting all your weight to one leg, like when putting on pants, can be another classic sign. If your hip pain is not improving or you suspect a pelvic stress fracture, go see a sports medicine doctor ASAP!

Happy Hips: Proper Hygiene, Rehab, and Prehab

We've gone through how the hip is designed to work and common injuries that can occur at the hip joint if the body is compensating or the hip isn't working or moving correctly. So what can be done to prevent problems from happening? How do we keep our hips mobile and strong?

The number one thing that we encourage when it comes to hip health is to adopt a daily hip mobility routine. We refer to this as *hip hygiene*. For runners, hip mobility exercises should be as routine as brushing and flossing your teeth every day! Especially with the computer-oriented universe most of us live in, we simply don't get enough movement throughout the day to keep this critical joint healthy.

Combining mobility with strength is critical to hip health. Strength will help your body make use of and maintain your mobility gains. First we cover the best mobility exercises for runners, and then we describe some valuable strength exercises.

Mobility Exercises

Many exercises will improve your hip strength and range of motion. The ones highlighted in this section are the most useful for runners.

Foam Rolling the Glutes, TFL, and Quads

Begin with foam rolling, which promotes tissue extensibility in a specific region, warming it up for movement. Foam roll the glutes, tensor fasciae latae (TFL), and quads.

Glutes: To foam roll the glutes, sit on a foam roller and cross one leg over the other (figure 8.3a). Slowly work your way over the muscle, paying specific attention to any areas that feel tender or knotty. Note if any areas seem to twitch or feel spastic. If you hit one of these trigger points, pause and sustain pressure for a few moments. You can incorporate deep breathing and active movements by slowly rocking your hips side to side, moving your knee like a windshield wiper, or bending and straightening the knee. Target the areas along the bony prominences and the tailbone. For a deeper release, you can try using a lacrosse ball, but be careful; it is possible to overdo it with a lacrosse ball, especially if the area is acutely irritated.

TFL/gluteus medius: For this technique, place the foam roller on your side, right below the top of your hip bone (figure 8.3*b*). The best way to do this is to lie on your side, prop yourself on one arm, and stack your top leg over your bottom leg, so you can use your top leg to support and stabilize as you roll the bottom hip. Work up and down this muscle, pausing on any areas that feel particularly tender. You can bend your bottom knee back and forth or rotate side to side for an active release. Work through the fleshy area from the top of your hip bone down to where your glute meets the top of your leg.

Quads: Lie on your abdomen, propped up on your forearms. Place the foam roller under one quad; brace the other leg up and out to the side to stabilize your position (figure 8.3*c*). We recommend breaking the quad into three sections: outer quad, along the IT band; middle quad; and inner quad, near the adductors. You can reach these sections by rotating your foot inward or outward, respectively. Begin with the foam roller right above your knee. Slowly roll your way up, inch by inch. If you find a spot that feels particularly knotty or tender, pause and sustain the pressure, taking three to five deep breaths, and bend your knee back and forth or side to side (like a windshield wiper). Repeat until you've worked your way through the whole muscle group.

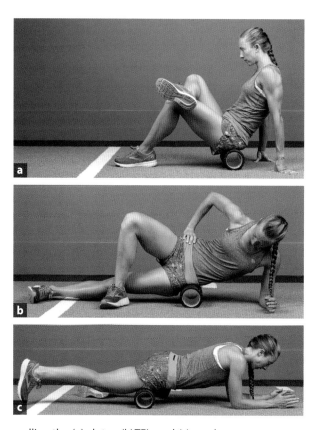

Figure 8.3 Foam rolling the *(a)* glutes, *(b)* TFL, and *(c)* quads.

Trigger Point Release: Hip Flexor (Psoas)

For this exercise, you'll need a lacrosse ball or something of similar size and density; a tennis ball can be a good and less intense start. Lie on your abdomen and place the ball right above your anterior superior iliac spine (ASIS, the bony projection of the iliac bone; figure 8.4) so the ball can access the inside of your pelvis. Take three to five deep breaths. Straighten your leg back and forth by flexing your toes or bending your knees.

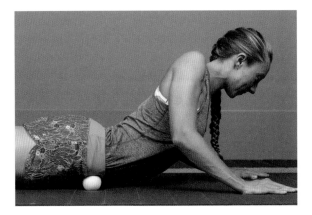

Figure 8.4   Trigger point release: hip flexor.

Hip Floss

The goal of hip flossing is to move the femur in the hip socket 360 degrees and move the pelvis around on the femur. You're teaching the brain to do these motions independently. This helps increase relative motion at the hip joint, which also helps to decrease compensatory patterns such as moving too much from the spine or lower leg. Another benefit of hip flossing is to hydrate the joint by redistributing fluid, break up soft tissue and fascial restrictions that lead to stiffness, and activate the deep hip muscles that both stabilize and move the hip.

Femur on pelvis: The goal of this exercise is to independently disassociate the femur from the pelvis by keeping the hip bones (pelvis) very still while moving the leg in all three planes of motion at the hip joint. This can be performed either standing while holding onto a wall or table for balance or on all fours. Bring the knee up and forward into flexion (figure 8.5a), then out to the side into abduction (figure 8.5b). Internally rotate the femur so the heel points toward the ceiling (figure 8.5c). Finally, bring the hip down and around into extension. Repeat five times clockwise, then reverse: extension, external rotation, adduction, and flexion. Perform the movements slowly and with control.

Pelvis on femur: This exercise can be a little trickier. We recommend propping one leg (the one you aren't moving) up on a small stool. Drive your hips forward so you feel a stretch in the front of your hip bone (figure 8.6a). Then, shift them medially into adduction, stretching the medial hip (figure 8.6b). Next, bring your hips around and back for posterior mobilization (figure 8.6c). Finally, move your hips laterally to the side, and then back to the front. Repeat five times clockwise and five times counterclockwise.

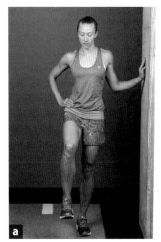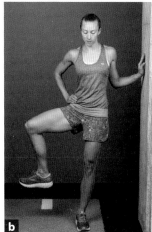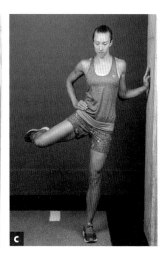

Figure 8.5   Hip floss, femur on pelvis: *(a)* start position; *(b)* leg to the side; *(b)* leg back.

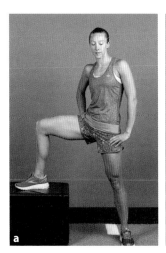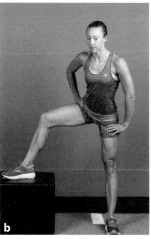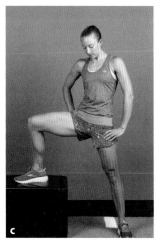

Figure 8.6   Hip floss, pelvis on femur: *(a)* start position; *(b)* pelvis back; *(c)* pelvis forward.

3D Pivots

This exercise is like WD-40 for the hip. Unlike hip flossing, the focus is not on moving the hip joint in isolation, but on engaging the whole kinetic chain to promote three-dimensional movement throughout the body, using the pelvis as the fulcrum.

Start by stepping forward and backward with one leg, alternating between hip flexion and hip extension (sagittal plane; figure 8.7, *a* and *b*) by following the moving leg with the hips. The stance leg is the focus; keep the leg and knee relatively straight, and focus on the movement at the pelvis. Repeat five times, then switch legs.

Next step side to side, or in the frontal plane, with one foot. Switch between abduction (figure 8.7*c*) and adduction (figure 8.7*d*), alternating between crossing the midline of the body with the moving foot and then stepping out into a side lunge, all while moving the inner and outer hip. Be careful not to compensate by twisting. Repeat five times, and then switch legs.

Last is rotation, or movement in the transverse plane. Alternate between internal and external rotation around a fixed foot (figure 8.7, *e* and *f*). Be careful your standing foot doesn't twist with you; try to center the movement at the pelvis. Step one foot (the moving foot) in front of the other, making a T shape with your feet. Feel the outside of the hip stretch as you twist internally, toward the unmoving stance leg. Then, rotate out so your feet make an L (or a backward L) shape. The inner thigh should stretch as you rotate externally. Repeat five times, and then switch legs.

3D pivots learned from Gray Institute®, GrayInstitute.com.

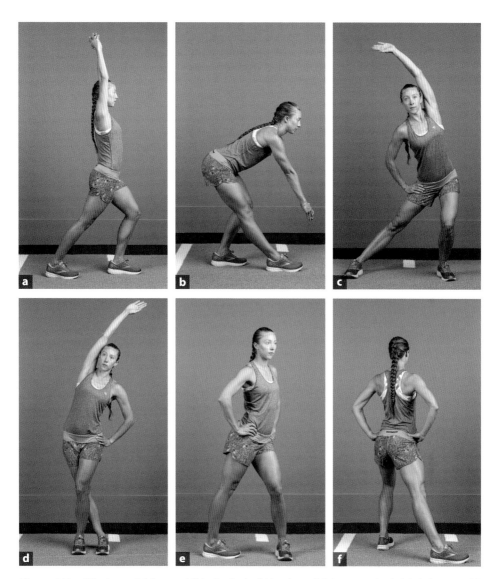

Figure 8.7 3D pivots: *(a)* forward (hip flexion); *(b)* backward (hip extension); *(c)* abduction; *(d)* adduction; *(e)* internal rotation; *(f)* external rotation.

Common Lunge Matrix

Again, here we are emphasizing triplanar hip movement, driving movement from the pelvis. Use this exercise prerun as a mobility warm-up, or, once you've mastered the movements, grab some dumbbells and repeat three sets of 10 as part of a strength-building routine.

Traditional forward lunge: These will be familiar. Lunge forward, keeping your weight in your front heel (figure 8.8a and figure 8.8b). Sink back into your hip. You should not feel strain in your knee or low back. For a more advanced version, keep your weight through your heel and use your glute to propel you up to balance on the lunging leg.

Lateral (side) lunge: This time, your lunging leg will move in the transverse plane, away from your body and to the side (figure 8.9). Make sure your knee doesn't go out too far; you want your hip, knee, and foot to all stay in alignment. For increased difficulty, use your glute to propel you up into a standing position on the lunging leg.

Rotational lunge: For this lunge, your lunging leg rotates away from your stance leg, so your feet form a very wide L shape (figure 8.10). Sink into your hip on the lunging leg. To progress, propel yourself up into a standing position on the lunging leg.

(For each of these lunges, bonus points if you are able to keep your lunging leg perfectly stable and rotate your pelvis toward that leg without your knee moving—you will need to engage your adductor slightly with an inward force to keep your knee steady.)

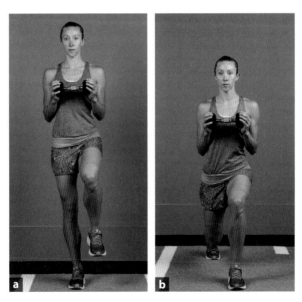

Figure 8.8   Common lunge matrix: traditional forward lunge. Figure 8.8a is also the start position for the subsequent two lunges.

Common lunge matrix learned from Gray Institute®, GrayInstitute.com.

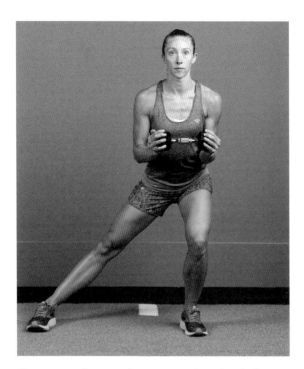

Figure 8.9   Common lunge matrix: lateral (side) lunge.

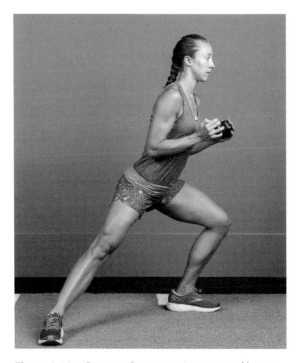

Figure 8.10   Common lunge matrix: rotational lunge.

Deep Squat

We love the deep squat. It's the position in which the body was designed to rest (and to eliminate waste). It also relaxes and lengthens your pelvic floor muscles, a muscle group that is commonly tight and overworked in runners. Yet we see many clients who lack the mobility and flexibility needed to deep squat, which has serious impacts on the health of the hip joint, low back, and pelvic floor. It can even contribute to gastrointestinal issues. To perform this exercise, simply drop down all the way to the ground so that your bottom is resting between your legs (figure 8.11). Hold for three to five breaths before returning to standing. Do 1 to 10 reps two or three times a day.

If you have trouble dropping into a deep squat, try using a door frame, counter, pole, or anything sturdy to assist. It may help to spread your legs wider or elevate your heels, since limitations in ankle mobility can affect the hips.

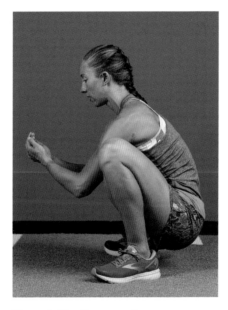

Figure 8.11   Deep squat.

Posterior Capsule Stretch

This stretch is similar to a pigeon pose, but it targets the joint capsule more specifically. The purpose of this stretch is to increase the range of motion in the back of the hip, which makes it easier to load the glutes and helps to decompress muscles such as the piriformis and other deep hip muscles that lead to issues such as sciatica, sacroiliac joint pain, and many other overuse issues at the hip.

Stand at a table or other surface approximately hip height. Place your leg on the table with your knee bent. (The stretch is easiest when the foot is closer to the thigh. The more you extend the lower leg toward a 90-degee angle, the deeper and more intense the stretch becomes.) Try to keep the knee directly in front of your hip (figure 8.12a). Then turn your body toward the leg on the table, initiating the movement with your pelvis, not your low back, and bring your arms over to the side. Bend your trunk toward the leg on the table (figure 8.12b) and rise slightly (no need to return all the way to starting position), being sure to keep your body turned toward the front leg. Repeat 5 to 10 times, then switch legs.

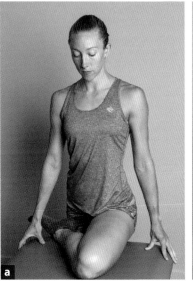 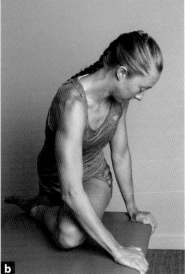

Figure 8.12   Posterior capsule stretch: *(a)* starting position; *(b)* stretch.

Strength Exercises

Strengthening the hip joint in all three planes of motion is necessary, even for runners. Just as you need to be able to move the hip in all three planes, you also need to be able to control the movement in all three planes. While running is primarily a forward-moving sport, components of the stride include side-to-side and rotational movement, so building resilience through these planes by strengthening the glutes, hamstrings, and quads is critical. Strength training should look like the sport of running when possible. Therefore, we recommend single-leg exercises, lunges, and drills that promote elastic recoil throughout the region.

Resisted Hip Isometrics

Runners often ignore the ability to control muscles through the end range of movement. A hip exercise that can be a game changer in reducing pain and injury risk is end-range resisted isometric contraction with core control to ensure that you're firing the muscle in the most advantageous position. There are six different resisted hip movements you can practice. This is also a great exercise to incorporate when returning to sport from an injury, as it activates all the muscles surrounding the hip so the joint is primed and ready for action.

Stand and face a wall, with your hands on the wall for balance. Tuck your hips, exhale, and make sure your deep abs are engaged to stabilize your pelvis. Then perform flexion, extension, abduction, adduction, internal rotation, and external rotation to strengthen the hip in all planes of motion.

For flexion, march one leg up as high as you can (figure 8.13*a*). You can use your hand to try to pull the leg higher. Hold this position for 5 to 10 seconds. To add resistance, use your free hand to push down against the leg, essentially fighting yourself. Repeat with the other leg.

For extension, bend one knee and punch that heel back and up toward the ceiling (figure 8.13*b*). Keep your core engaged, and don't arch your low back; you should feel your glute working. Hold for 5 to 10 seconds, and repeat with the other leg.

For abduction, lift your knee up to 90 degrees, or as high as you comfortably can, and rotate that leg out to the side (figure 8.13*c*). Continue to brace your core. Hold for 5 to 10 seconds. (You can also use your hand to add resistance.) Repeat with the other leg.

For adduction, lift your knee up to 90 degrees, or as high as you comfortably can, and pull the leg across your body as far as you can (figure 8.13*d*). You can use your hand to pull the leg farther or add resistance, if you like. Hold for 5 to 10 seconds, and repeat with the other leg.

For internal rotation, lift your leg up to 90 degrees, or as high as you comfortably can, and then rotate your heel toward your midline (figure 8.13*e*). Hold for 5 to 10 seconds, and repeat with the other leg.

For external rotation, lift your leg up to 90 degrees, or as high as you comfortably can, and rotate your heel away from your midline (figure 8.13*f*). Hold for 5 to 10 seconds, and repeat with the other leg. (For added strength gains, work to increase the hold to 30 seconds or up to 1 minute.)

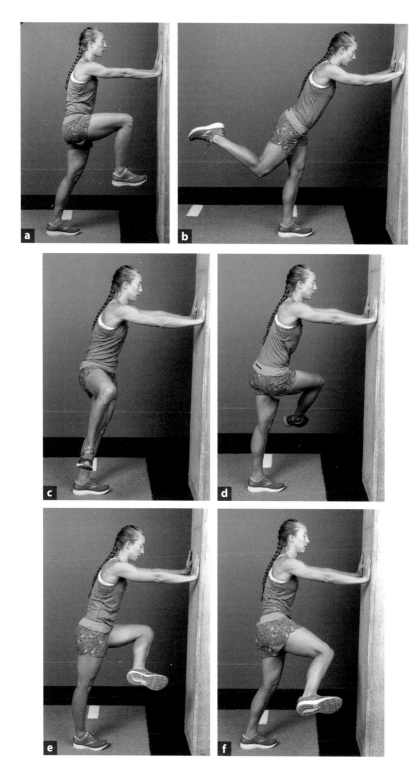

Figure 8.13   Resisted hip isometrics: *(a)* flexion; *(b)* extension; *(c)* abduction; *(d)* adduction; *(e)* internal rotation; *(f)* external rotation.

Standing Hip Internal Rotation Lunge

Stand in a staggered stance (figure 8.14a). Shift your weight onto the front heel. Rotate toward your front hip, keeping your knee pointed straight forward (figure 8.14b). You should feel a stretch in the back, not the side, of your hip. Return to the starting position. Repeat 10 times on each leg. This promotes proper posterior loading of the glute and hip joint capsule, as discussed earlier in the chapter.

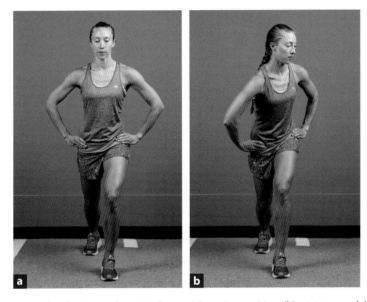

Figure 8.14   Standing hip internal rotation lunge: (a) starting position; (b) rotate toward the front hip.

Core Stability

Incorporating core stability training into your routine is also key. For running, the core needs to remain stable as the pelvis moves. A great exercise to start with is the all-four belly lift (detailed in chapter 9). Progressing core strength to include dynamic movements teaches the body to stabilize with the core while moving the lower limbs, the way we want it to function in everyday life and especially when running. We recommend the plank with hip drivers, outlined in chapter 9. Strengthening your core in proper alignment wards off injuries like impingement and groin pain because it emphasizes a neutral pelvis, which promotes the femur functioning from the proper position. A weak core is a common underlying cause for tight hips—if the body isn't getting the proper stability from the core, it will be quick to compensate with surrounding muscle groups.

Good Running Form

The glutes, abdominal muscles, hip flexors, and quads all work together for an efficient stride. The gluteus medius plays a critical role in pelvic stability when landing and switching from one leg to the other, while the gluteus maximus is a power driver that works in conjunction with the obliques to effectively propel you forward. This is important when increasing speeds because it is how we maintain a full gait cycle and avoid compensatory strategies like excessive low back torque or reliance on quads or calves (Lenhart, Thelen, and Heiderscheit 2014).

Another thing to be hip-mindful of when running is maintaining a forward lean from the ankle up. Maintaining a forward angle not only reduces your workload (in this posture, gravity is *helping* you, versus a more upright posture, where you are fighting it), it also aligns you in a position where it is biomechanically easier to use your glutes than your quads. A more upright or "seated" posture in running puts more stress on your knee extensors or quads; instead of propelling forward, you are pulling your leg forward. Over time, this causes a jamming of the hip joint and a lack of posterior motion of the femur into the pelvis, which prevents the glutes from loading (Teng and Powers 2016).

Case Study: Martha

Martha presents with pain in her hip that is worse after running but hard to pinpoint.
Observation: Upon inspection, she has limited rotation in her hip joint, as well as increased dynamic valgus on loading.
Diagnosis: Labral tear (confirmed by MRI).
Treatment: Martha is given a meticulous home mobility routine to perform before runs (in line with what is listed in the mobility section of this chapter), as well as hip flexor mobility and gluteus medius and gluteus maximus strengthening stabilization exercises. She is ultimately able to return to running pain-free with the addition of her at-home exercises.

Case Study: Sofia

Sofia presents with a labral tear, which was diagnosed by her doctor prior to beginning treatment.
Observation: Sofia's symptoms stem from tight, overdominant quads that prevent her from being able to load posteriorly into her hip joint to engage her glutes.
Diagnosis: Labral tear.
Treatment: Sofia is given mobility exercises to work on hip internal rotation and posterior capsule stretching and is taught to practice sinking deeper into her hip joint with strength training, posture, and loading exercises. This is paired with deep core and glute strengthening exercises to promote increased pelvic stability when landing. This increased posterior joint mobility allows Sofia to better access her glutes in order to off-load her quads. Sofia has also not had any significant flare-ups of pelvic pain since.

Conclusion

Hip injury is multifaceted and interconnected. By understanding how the joint is designed to move and function in running, you can get to the root cause of hip injuries and prevent them from occurring.

CHAPTER 9

Low Back

Much of this book covers what can go wrong in the lower extremities when the pelvis locks up and the glute muscles aren't working well. Now we shift our focus up the chain to the low back. Although some people believe that the impact of running is bad for the low back, there is evidence that running can be protective of the low back. On average, runners are less likely to have low back pain than the normal population (Maselli et al. 2020). However, bad form while running can adversely affect your low back and lead to back pain. This chapter delves into why this happens and what you can do to prevent it.

To understand injury in the low back of a runner, we must first understand how the low back is intended to function when we run. Like in most activities, our body's core and low back help us maintain stability (i.e., staying upright, fighting gravity, not falling over), while our extremities above and below the core are rapidly moving. In addition to stabilization, this central region must protect vulnerable parts of our bodies.

A runner generates forward propulsion primarily via the reciprocal rotational movement between the pelvis (powered by the glutes) and the thoracic spine (powered by the obliques) (figure 9.1). These two regions of the body work together, in opposition, by rotating to create torque that helps a runner smoothly progress forward. In between these two rotating structures lies the lumbar spine (the low back), our abdominal muscles, and all our internal organs.

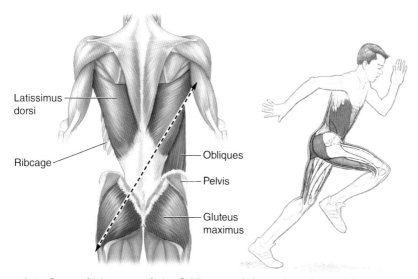

Figure 9.1 Power-driving cross-chain of obliques and glutes plus pelvic and thoracic spine rotation.

Runners need enough mobility and strength in their pelvis and upper body to propel forward efficiently, essentially by creating reciprocating slingshots between the obliques and the glutes. Runners also must move with good alignment so that the core stability muscles can function as intended.

Core as a Can

Just as the design of a can functions as a pressure control (keeping that soda or beer perfectly carbonated), our body's core functions similarly. We have our diaphragm on top, which, besides controlling our breathing, acts as the top of our can of muscles (figure 9.2). Our abdominal muscles in the front wrap around to connect with our lumbar stabilizers in the back, protecting our abdominal cavity on all sides. At the bottom, our pelvic floor muscles support our urogenital organs and help to stabilize the lower spine and pelvis. Keeping the ribs and the pelvis stacked, or aligned well, is vital for proper pressure control—and good running mechanics.

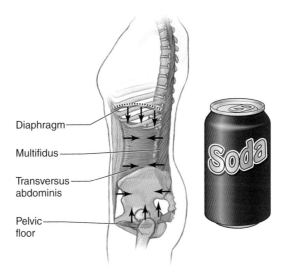

Figure 9.2   The importance of proper alignment for pressure control—your *core can*.

Finally, if our core is meant to mimic a can, it's important that the ribs and pelvis are lined up rather than hyperextended (or overly slouched), which is a posture toward which many runners gravitate.

Etiology of Low Back Injury

When dysfunction exists between the thoracic spine and the pelvis, the low back gets caught in the middle. Restrictions in the pelvis or thoracic spine can limit efficient transfer of power through the core. These restrictions often cause excessive forces to go through the lumbar spine, leading to low back pain in runners. This area can get grossly overworked, causing pain and spasm in the low back muscles, and can lead to injury in the spine itself. If low back issues are not properly addressed, early problems can lead to more significant damage, such as disc herniations, spinal stenosis, or pain that radiates down the leg, affecting the use of the lower extremity.

Adequate rotation through the pelvis helps you properly load the hip and recruit the glutes for forward propulsion. The pelvis must be able to move forward and backward (anteriorly and posteriorly) as we transition from stance leg to swing leg in our gait. Restrictions in the front of the hip, or hip flexors that are too tight, limit the ability of the femur to extend backward on the pelvis. This causes the pelvis to stay "stuck" in an anteriorly rotated position. Think of the position your hips are in when you are sitting in a chair. Then, imagine standing up, but your hips stay stuck in that position.

Runners often compensate for poor hip extension by extending their low back to orient the upper part of the body straight against gravity. This leads to a hyperlordosis, or overextension, of the lumbar spine. So the human body can fight gravity, maintain balance, and function upright, the ribs also rotate upward and the entire front of our postural chain acts in an overlengthened and expanded position. This prevents us from getting adequate stability from our abdominal muscles and generating power through our obliques.

Where do we turn for muscular strength instead? We recruit the low back (and sometimes our hip flexors, too). In addition to supporting the runner's torso, the low back muscles also function as hip extensors. When the pelvis is rotated forward, the glutes aren't able to work properly to extend the femur on the pelvis, so instead, the runner compensates by gaining extra extension (push-off) from the low back, further exacerbating the problem.

One of the most common mistakes that runners make is running overly upright. Running instructions are often "stand tall," "chest up," "chest forward," but the extreme version of this can be just as detrimental as running in an overly slouched position. When a runner stands up too straight, it causes an increased rib flare, meaning the chest becomes oriented up and out (figure 9.3*a* and figure 9.3*b*). This drives dysfunction in the back; now we have overstretched and overlengthened abdominal muscles, overworked low back muscles, and a spine in a disadvantageous position to rotate.

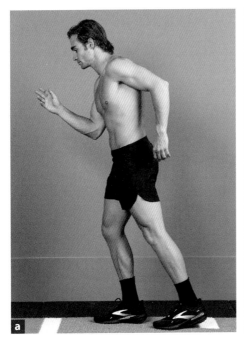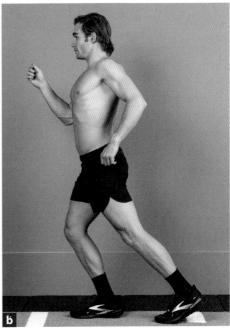

Figure 9.3   *(a)* Proper alignment and core function versus *(b)* hyperextension.

Injury Specifics

Now that we have a better understanding of what can go wrong with the low back, let's delve a little bit deeper into the pathology of specific injuries. It isn't at all uncommon for the low back muscles to become tight, fatigued, and overworked due to the compensatory patterns to which we often fall victim. Aside from general soreness, overuse, and muscle strain, the joints of the spine can also be affected. This is usually a sharp, intense injury that can be confusing for a runner.

Facet Syndrome

Acutely, inflammation and irritation can occur within the joints of the spine or at the spine and pelvis juncture. Some common resultant injuries are labeled *facet syndrome* or *sacroiliac joint dysfunction*. The common denominator of these injuries is irritation in the joint itself—inflammation that exists between the bones. This happens when there's too much motion in a place there shouldn't be. Sometimes, we even get some bone-on-bone friction, which can create a sharp, intense pain that can take several weeks to resolve. The more we can mobilize, stabilize, and strengthen the muscles around the pelvis and spine, the less likely facet syndrome is to occur.

Case Study: Mariana

Mariana presents to physical therapy with complaints of low back pain during and after her long runs; she reports that her back doesn't tend to hurt on her shorter runs. The pain seems to last for a couple days and affects her day-to-day activities, like driving in her car or sitting for extended periods at work.

Observation: Upon evaluation, Mariana demonstrates decreased hip rotation bilaterally. When standing, she has an anterior pelvic tilt. She hyperextends her low back when she runs, and the result is increased rotation through her low back with decreased scapula and thoracic spine movement. She is also limited in her hip extension; with decreased glute strength and increased muscle definition and tightness in her lumbar paraspinals.

Diagnosis: Postural syndrome; without intervention, her condition could progress to spondylosis (hyperextension left untreated that causes the forward slippage of the discs).

Treatment: Treatment consists of postural reeducation, specifically cueing Mariana to exhale, lean forward, and drop her ribs down when she runs. This is combined with hip mobilization and deep core strengthening to allow Mariana to maintain good form while she runs and not fatigue into faulty mechanics. After treatment, Mariana reports she now feels like she can sustain proper form better. She has become aware of when she starts to fatigue and hyperextend, so she is able to exhale and restore herself to proper form.

Herniated Disc

Runners are more prone to spine and disc injury when the muscles in the low back are overworked, fatigued, or weak—such as when abdominal stabilizing muscles aren't able to do their job to stabilize the spine—or when there are restrictions in our joints. The pain of a herniated disc is usually localized but can sometimes radiate down one or both legs. Usually, avoiding impact activities for a few days and performing gentle movement and strength work will help resolve the pain, but sometimes the inflammation in the disc can cause nerve problems or pain that radiates into the extremities. If you are experiencing any new onset of muscle weakness, go to your doctor as soon as possible.

Red Flags

If you've ever been formally diagnosed with a herniated disc or spinal stenosis, even though it doesn't mean that you necessarily should not run we recommend working with a skilled physical therapist on proper form, mechanics, and strengthening exercises to reduce your chances of re-exacerbating this injury. This book cannot replace hands-on physical therapy. Additionally, if you have pain that radiates down the leg or feel burning, tingling, or numbness, it could be a sign that you have nerve involvement. Finally, if you feel like you have a new onset of weakness in your leg (often but not always concurrent with low back pain), see a doctor as soon as possible.

Treatment

If you have low back pain, the first step is identifying if tightness, weakness, or some combination of the two is causing your pain. We break down treatment into four categories: upper back and thoracic spine tightness, core muscle weakness, hip tightness, and hip weakness. If you're unsure where to start, chances are you could benefit from addressing the upper back (thoracic spine) and the pelvis.

Upper Back and Thoracic Spine Tightness

Limitations in thoracic spine mobility are extremely common, especially in people with desk jobs. If you're reading this and thinking "I've been this way forever," that's even more reason to work on your mobility, because a little bit of attention can go a long way.

Here are a few exercises that can help to improve your thoracic spine mobility.

Foam Roll Thoracic Spine

Lie on your back with your hands behind your head and a foam roller lengthwise below your mid- to upper back (figure 9.4a). Choose areas of focus along the shoulder blades—such as just below, in the middle, and just above—and adjust based on where you feel stiff or restricted. Remember to stay on the part of your back where you have ribs (hence the shoulder blade guidance).

Balance your shoulders over the foam roller into extension (lean back) (figure 9.4b). This should feel like a very good stretch; you might even get a couple pops. Curl back up, and then extend back again, three or four times.

Next, rock your shoulders and elbows from side to side to facilitate transverse plane movement (figure 9.4c). Finally, do three clockwise and three counterclockwise arm circles (figure 9.4d).

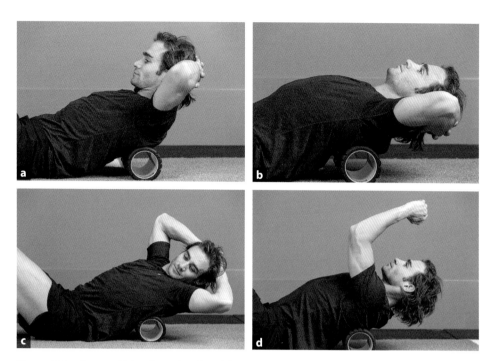

Figure 9.4   Foam roll the thoracic spine: *(a)* starting position; *(b)* lean back; *(c)* rotation; *(d)* arm circles.

Thread the Needle

Begin on your hands and knees. Reach one arm to the ceiling, rotating as high up as you can, opening the chest (figure 9.5*a*). Lower it toward the floor, and reach your arm through the space between your standing arm and knee as far as you can (figure 9.5*b*), stretching the back of the thoracic cavity. Repeat 10 times each side.

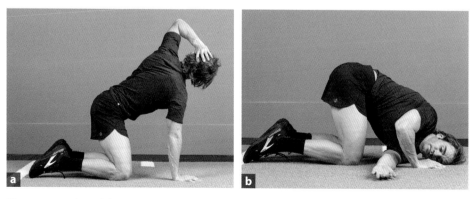

Figure 9.5   Thread the needle: *(a)* reach up; *(b)* reach through.

3D Arm Matrix

Fix one arm on a desk or table or just hold it still. The other arm will lead the thoracic spine into all three planes of motion. First, swing your arm up and overhead, and then down and back (figure 9.6, *a* and *b*). Don't be afraid to make the movements big. Going a little bit faster and getting some momentum behind you can help. Repeat this 5 to 10 times. Next, reach your arm up and over your head toward your other side, and then down (side bend), driving your elbow into your side (figure 9.6, *c* and *d*). Also repeat 5 to 10 times. Finally, reach across your body and forward, feeling the shoulder muscles engage a little bit, and then backward, drawing your shoulder blade with you (figure 9.6, *e* and *f*). Perform 5 to 10 times. Switch arms.

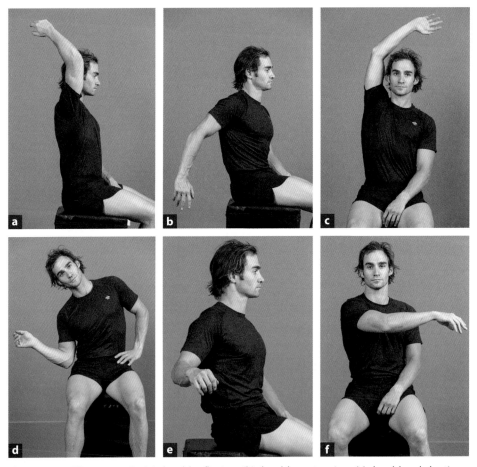

Figure 9.6   3D arm matrix: *(a)* shoulder flexion; *(b)* shoulder extension; *(c)* shoulder abduction; *(d)* shoulder adduction; *(e)* horizontal abduction; *(f)* horizontal adduction.

3D arm matrix learned from Gray Institute®, GrayInstitute.com.

Runner's Lunge With Focus on Arm Drive

This exercise integrates upper and lower body mechanics. Stand with your feet in a staggered stance (imagine you are running). We are practicing swinging the arms and shoulders back and forth. Keeping your eyes up and ahead and your feet, knees, and hips very still, think about reaching your arm forward on one side while the other shoulder and elbow are pushing backward (figure 9.7a). You should feel the muscles in the front of your shoulder and the back of your shoulder activate as you do this. You can try adding some hand weights to this exercise; see if you can feel your obliques kicking in with heavier weights.

To advance this exercise, practice coming up to balance on the stance leg as you rotate your arms, engaging your glutes and obliques simultaneously (figure 9.7b).

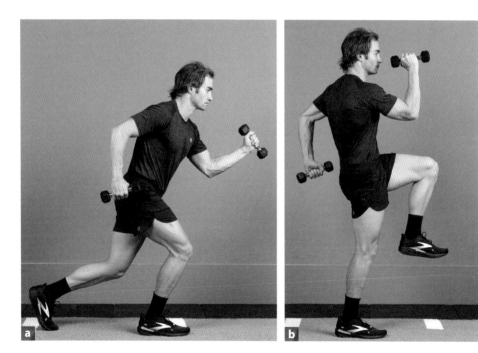

Figure 9.7   Runner's lunge with focus on arm drive: *(a)* leg down; *(b)* leg up.

Core Muscle Weakness

Talk to anyone about low back pain and the first thing they'll mention is core strength. So what exactly is the purpose of core strength, and how can it help? Thoracic spine rotation facilitated by the obliques is one of the major components of running, so having adequate oblique strength helps to reduce compensatory low back rotation (Raabe and Chaudhari 2018). Strong deep abdominal stabilizers provide resistance to the rotational forces occurring above and below the low back during the running gait cycle. Having a strong "core can" (diaphragm, obliques, transversus abdominis, multifidus, and pelvic floor) helps to properly position the pelvis and ribs for maximum stability, creating a strong, dynamic core. This allows both the upper and lower extremities to function properly and can even contribute to helping with different types of gastrointestinal issues.

If you want to strengthen your core, first learn to identify and activate the different abdominal muscles, before doing further strength training.

Activation

Transversus abdominis: The transversus abdominis (TA) is a very important core muscle. The TA helps with digestion, posture, and pelvic floor control, and it keeps us upright while also protecting our low back. Due to habitual postures, breathing mechanics, trauma, or giving birth, this muscle can become very weak. A weak TA is a driving force behind low back pain and a whole host of other issues.

The best way to check if your TA is working properly is to lie on your back, put both hands on the inside of your hip bones, draw your belly button up, and let out a "shhhhh" sound; the muscle you feel contracting is your TA. It should be right under your fingertips, and you should feel a deep band across your low abs. Hold the contraction for 5 to 10 breaths. This is activation and isolation. We will get into functional movements shortly.

Obliques: To isolate the obliques, try a side plank (figure 9.8). Lie on your side with your knees bent, propped up onto your elbow, and push up into a side plank. Reach your top arm forward, so your torso is rotated a little bit toward the ground and you feel a stretch in your upper back. Try to stack the pelvis and ribs.

Multifidus: The multifidus is a posterior chain muscle that is also critical for spinal stabilization. To activate this muscle, sit or stand at a desk or table. With your hands in fists, push on the table from underneath the table (figure

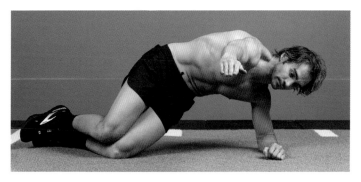

Figure 9.8   Side plank.

9.9). You should feel muscles in your back turn on; the multifidus is engaged. This is a great exercise to do during the day at work.

Diaphragm: It's pretty challenging to isolate and activate your diaphragm muscle, but you can feel confident that if your abdominal, spinal stabilizing, and pelvic floor muscles are engaging and you have good alignment between your ribs and pelvis, your diaphragm is in good shape to function properly.

Pelvic floor: This critical muscle group—composed of 12 different muscles—is often overlooked but plays a critical role in core stability and protecting the low back from injury. If you have suboptimal use of any of the previously described core muscles, you are more likely to have a pelvic floor that is functioning in either a hypertonic (overactive, making up for abdominal weakness) or hypotonic (underactive, unable to properly stabilize and fire) state, which can be a big driver of injury. If you've ever experienced any urinary or bowel incontinence, pain with sex or tampon insertion, or symptoms that haven't responded to other treatment methods, pelvic floor dysfunction could be an underlying reason.

Rectus abdominis: For runners, having a strong rectus abdominis, or six-pack muscle, is not that important. Why? This muscle is a fast twitch, sagittal plane muscle that is very useful when you're choking or expelling food from your body. (Essentially, it's your vomit muscle.) In running, an overdominant rectus abdominis can prevent proper rotational and cross-train (glutes and obliques working in reciprocal harmony) movement.

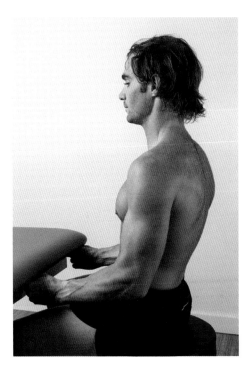

Figure 9.9 Multifidus activation.

Planks for Core Training

The simple activation and isolation exercises described in the previous section are a great place to start before graduating to more complex movements. We want to make sure that we can recruit these deeper muscles with proper alignment and positioning to better stabilize the spine before practicing global and functional movements.

Another exercise to practice consistently is the plank; it is the most functional way to train your core. We've evolved from quadruped animals whose core muscles were almost constantly being recruited for just about all activities. On all fours, the abs are constantly resisting gravity, being used in gait, and more.

Before getting into a basic plank, we recommend you start with the all-four belly lift. This is another great way to activate your core, and it promotes healthy alignment (keeping your ribs and hips stacked).

All-Four Belly Lift

Start on your hands and knees. Rock your hips back and forth a few times (if you've done yoga, this is often called *cat/cow*), and then try to find the middle between these two—pelvic neutral. If you aren't quite sure where your pelvic neutral position is, a slight tuck is okay, too. Next, press your hands firmly into the ground, drawing your sternum up toward the ceiling; you should feel your shoulders engage (serratus). Rock your nose forward so it is just past your fingertips (this activates your transversus abdominis). Hold this position, and finally, lift your knees off the ground, just about an inch (figure 9.10). Now, hold for five breaths. On your inhale, focus on sending the air into your back and keeping your back and pelvis still; don't let yourself rock forward. On your exhale, focus on drawing your ribs down and in, pulling them toward your pelvis. If this is too hard, you can start by keeping your knees on the ground as you practice these breaths and eventually progress to lifting them off the floor.

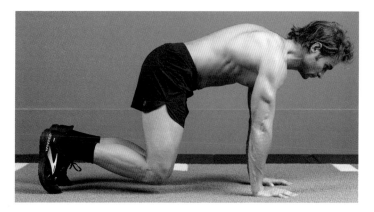

Figure 9.10   All-four belly lift.

This exercise can be progressed to a traditional plank (figure 9.11), but again, be sure to focus on keeping ribs and hips aligned and not overextending your back. Hold planks for a number of breaths, rather than a number of seconds, because the core is engaged through breathing.

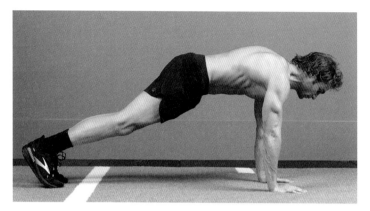

Figure 9.11   Traditional plank.

3D Plank With Hip Drivers

Rather than holding a static plank for minutes at a time, we want to train our core to function reactively, meaning that the abs work to stabilize as the pelvis, arms, and legs move. Therefore, adding triplanar movement to core exercises is useful.

Get into the traditional plank position, with two hands on the floor, arms straight, and shoulders stacked over your elbows, which are stacked over your wrists. Start by tilting your pelvis forward and backward, similar to cat/cow but with a flat back. You should feel those abs working to stabilize as your pelvis moves. Repeat 5 to 10 times. Next, move your hips side to side, keeping them parallel to the ground, like a dog wagging its tail. Repeat 5 to 10 times. Finally, add in rotation, or hip dips, coming back to neutral with each rotation. Start with 5 in each direction and work your way up to 10. For an added challenge, try using your leg or arm as the driver. You can move either extremity up and down, side to side, and rotationally.

Elbow-to-Knee Side Plank

Lie on your side, propped up on your elbow, and raise your hips to get into a side plank (figure 9.12a). (You can stagger your feet so the top leg is in front of the bottom leg for additional support.) Move your bottom knee and your top elbow toward your midline until they meet (figure 9.12b), accompanied with a strong exhale. That core should light up!

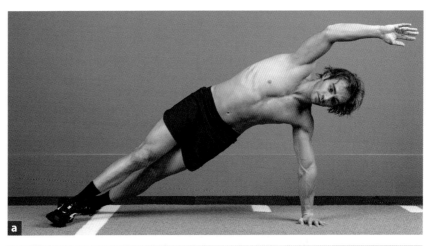

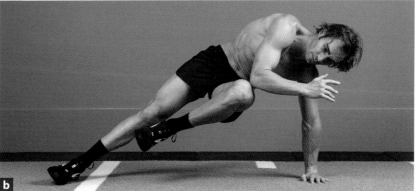

Figure 9.12   Elbow-to-knee side plank: *(a)* start position; *(b)* elbow to knee.

Hip Tightness

The factors discussed earlier can be driving forces for pelvic stiffness. Especially if you are dealing with a weak core or core that is functioning suboptimally, the body will turn to the hips for stability. Inversely, stiffness in the hips can lead to issues further up the chain. By now you should understand that hip tightness can lead to injury. A protocol similar to that discussed in previous chapters can be followed to allow for hip rotation during gait to reduce loading on the lumbar spine.

We also want to emphasize the importance of getting reciprocal rotation between the two halves of the pelvis when you run. If the pelvis, which is designed to be a primary rotator propelled by the glute muscles, isn't working properly, then the low back is quick to compensate to get the job done. This is why you align the ribs and pelvis and focus on turning from your hips while keeping your abs engaged, so that this excessive rotation does not come from the spine.

For details on how to work on hip mobility, turn to the hip mobility section of chapter 8.

Hip Weakness

Weakness in the glutes, hamstrings, and other muscles of the hip can cause compensations where the runner is seeking power and forward propulsion from the spine instead of from the proper muscles. In addition to undergoing mobility and gait retraining, strengthen the glutes and quads and work on functional running drills to tie all the pieces together. See the hip strength section of chapter 8 for a detailed explanation of hip strengthening exercises.

Other Treatment Considerations

A few additional (and more general) considerations to investigate if you are a runner dealing with low back pain are running shoes, running surface, and cadence. Old sneakers without enough support or cushioning can result in increased loading force through the low back. As with other injuries, logging lots of miles on concrete can also overstress the low back. Finally, just as overstriding can overstress the knee and hip joints, it can also cause excessive loading impact through the lumbar spine, especially if you have any preexisting conditions. Working with a coach or physical therapist on form and stride to help reduce the load and impact that you're placing on your low back can be a serious game changer.

Conclusion

This chapter explained some of the common causes of low back pain, which are connected to the upper back and the rest of the body. Back issues can also be reflected in other areas of the body, from the ankles to the neck. To avoid these issues, mobility and strength exercises for the back should be part of a runner's regular routine. See a professional if you cannot identify the source of any pain you're experiencing.

PART III

COMMON CONDITIONS

CHAPTER 10

Plantar Fasciitis

Plantar fasciitis is a cringeworthy tongue twister of a word and a common fear among runners—arch pain that can throw a wrench into your training, cause excruciating pain as you get out of bed in the morning, or leave you hobbling off the track after a workout. Yet before we get into the pain part, we need to understand what the plantar fascia is and does.

The plantar fascia is a dense connective tissue (*not* a muscle) whose role in running is to act as a lever arm that propels you forward. In technical terms, the plantar fascia is a ligament connecting your calcaneus to the other bones in your foot. It's responsible for helping the arch collapse as a loading response when you land (pronation) and then switching back to a rigid lever that propels you forward (supination) during push-off (McDonald et al. 2016).

Causes of Plantar Fasciitis

Plantar fasciitis, or inflammation of the plantar fascia (figure 10.1), is a finicky injury that can be frustrating to deal with. Too much movement (hypermobility) or too little movement (hypomobility) of the foot bones and plantar fascia can lead to pain, inflammation, and even tearing, in severe cases.

Tension in the calf can also play a big role in the development of plantar fasciitis, causing decreased mobility through the ankle and foot and making

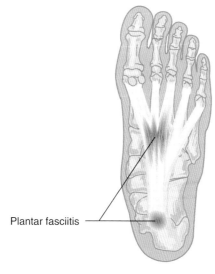

Plantar fasciitis

Figure 10.1   Plantar fasciitis.

a runner more susceptible to plantar fasciitis or Achilles tendinitis (which we will cover in the next chapter). The tissue that makes up the Achilles tendon is directly connected to the plantar fascia, and sometimes it can be almost a matter of chance which structure in the region is injured.

Diagnosis

Plantar fasciitis most commonly presents with pain at the insertion point of the plantar fascia—at the base of your heel bone, slightly toward the inside of your foot.

Although less common, you can still experience plantar fasciitis without insertional pain; in some instances it presents as tenderness or pain in the arch. Also, the plantar fascia shares some fibers with the posterior tibial tendon, so there can be some crossover between these two structures (or "itises"). Because of the shared fibers, getting a correct diagnosis can sometimes be tricky. For more information on ankle tendinitis, see chapter 6. It's possible to have both plantar fasciitis and posterior tibial tendinitis concurrently, so a collective treatment approach may be useful if that winds up being your diagnosis.

Symptoms of plantar fasciitis are typically worse in the morning—the hallmark symptom is acute pain with those first few steps out of bed. Usually, the pain will start to get better with activity or during a run, as the fascia and the muscle that attach to it loosen up, but then symptoms may worsen later in the day as the fascia cools down and starts to stiffen again. This is because of the type of connective tissue that makes up the plantar fascia. This dense connective tissue is slow to recover from the load and stress placed on it during effort or exertion. This makes the plantar fascia prone to inflammation.

Inflammation is inherently a good thing; it's the way that the tissues in our body respond to different forces placed on them—by adapting to grow stronger. Where we run into trouble is when we don't allow enough time for the tissue to adapt between efforts and we are inflaming tissue that is still recovering from our last exertion. The feet are especially tricky, because even when we are recovering between runs, we are still on our feet, going about our day. It's almost impossible to completely off-load this part of the body.

While plantar fasciitis can present in a number of different ways in the foot, keep in mind that this is not the only injury that can affect the foot. Other foot pain–causing injuries include an actual tear of your plantar fascia, a stress fracture, a small intrinsic foot muscle strain, a neuroma, or cuboid syndrome. (Remember: This book does not replace checking with your doctor, podiatrist, or physical therapist to get to the root of your injury.) Once you feel confident that what you are experiencing is, in fact, plantar fasciitis—inflammation of the plantar fascia—read on.

Hypermobile Versus Hypomobile Considerations

Generally, plantar fasciitis can be broken down into two major categories: a *hyper*mobile arch or a *hypo*mobile arch.

Traditionally, plantar fasciitis is associated with those who have a *hyper*mobile arch. *Hypermobility* is a term used to describe excess motion in a part of the body. A hypermobile arch presents with excessive pronation (arch collapse) during walking and running, which results in excessive stretching and overloading of the plantar fascia.

Alternatively, in the running population, it is not uncommon to see plantar fasciitis that is associated with a *hypomobile*, or more rigid, arch—an arch that *cannot* collapse. This results in restricted movement, a lack of blood flow, and an uneven distribution of impact forces through the tissue.

A runner with a flat foot, a foot that is very pronated, can still have a *hypo*mobile, or rigid, arch; pronation and hypermobility do not always go together. On the other hand, a runner with a high arch and supinated foot can still have a great degree of movement and mobility. What is key for a healthy, productive stride is that your foot can switch back and forth between pronation and supination efficiently as you move.

To treat plantar fasciitis properly, it's necessary to identify if your pain is being caused by hypermobility or hypomobility. In the following sections, we break down these two categories with examples of each and differences in treatment.

Hypermobile (Mobile) Plantar Fasciitis

If you are prone to wearing out the inside edges of your shoes (closest to your bellybutton, or midline), have difficulty activating your arch, or have general foot and ankle weakness or poor balance, you may have a *hypermobile* foot, which would place you in the arch-too-mobile category.

Hypomobile (Rigid) Plantar Fasciitis

If you are prone to really tight calves or notice a wear pattern on the outside edges of your running shoes (the edges closer to your shoulders than your bellybutton), chances are that you may not be getting enough movement through your foot. In addition to your natural biological structure, prior foot injuries can also contribute to having a more rigid foot, resulting in a compensatory, locked-up gait pattern.

Treatment and Prevention of Plantar Fasciitis

As we've explained, different factors can be at play in the root cause of plantar fasciitis. Consequently, treatments differ based on the underlying cause.

Case Study: Casey

Casey presents to physical therapy with pain in the arch of his foot that began after a 10-mile run a few weeks ago. Casey reports that the run was a bit longer than what he was used to, and some of the route was on more uneven terrain, so he isn't sure if that's what aggravated his foot or not. Casey reports that he took a few days off, iced his arch, and stretched his calf but has not seen any improvements in his symptoms.

Observation: When he walks, Casey has a strong inward roll of his ankle with every step he takes. When asked to stand on one foot, Casey's foot rolls inward, and he is unable to balance. The insides of his shoes are more worn than the outside, and when Casey runs, there is a lot of side-to-side movement of his hips.

Diagnosis: Hypermobile plantar fasciitis.

Treatment: In addition to soft tissue work to promote blood flow to the arch of the foot, treatment for Casey consists of arch-strengthening exercises (see chapter 5), glute- and hip-strengthening exercises (see chapters 7 and 8), and neuromuscular reeducation to train Casey to be able to engage his arch and glute together. Casey also benefits from wearing shoes with arch support to offload the plantar fascia and allow the inflamed area to heal before he begins his slow progression back to running.

Case Study: Alex

Alex presents to physical therapy with complaints of arch pain that began after a hard interval workout that he did a few weeks ago. Alex reports that despite resting his foot, icing it, and stretching his calves, he isn't noticing any improvement in his symptoms.

Observation: Alex's foot barely pronates when he walks. He also has trouble balancing and favors the outside of his foot for stability. When Alex runs, he bounces a lot, with over-recruitment of his calves, and he lands on the outside of his foot; there is little movement through his ankle.

Diagnosis: Hypomobile plantar fasciitis.

Treatment: Alex's physical therapist performs manual work to release tension in the arch and bottom of his foot, mobilize his calcaneus and arch, and facilitate ankle pronation. Treatment also includes exercises to dynamically stretch out the calf, exercises to increase pronation and efficacy with proper joint loading, and cueing to relax his arches and land on the inside of his foot while walking and running. Initially, Alex is advised to wear supportive footwear during all weight-bearing activity in order to off-load the plantar fascia and promote healing, but as his symptoms resolve Alex is encouraged to work his way back to being able to tolerate barefoot loading for increased increments of time. Athletic kinesiology tape is also used to increase Alex's proprioceptive awareness of letting his arch relax when standing and walking.

In the case of hypermobility, you'll want to strengthen the muscles of the foot to reduce the excessive loading of the plantar fascia. This can be achieved through activation of the intrinsic foot muscles and the arch. See chapter 5 for appropriate exercises.

In the case of hypomobility, focus the treatment on loosening up and relaxing the arch to help increase mobility throughout the foot. This can be achieved through a number of exercises. Techniques for splaying your feet and the pronation driver exercise can be found in chapter 5, and the three-way calf stretch and foam and ball rolling for the calf can be found in chapter 6.

Depending on how acute your injury is, you may benefit from wearing supportive footwear to lessen the strain that's being put on the plantar fascia. This will never be a permanent solution for plantar fasciitis, but in the short term it can help allow the inflammation to settle down. If you are experiencing sharp pain when walking, especially if it's causing you to limp or causing pain in other parts of your foot, you probably fall into this category. Birkenstock-type sandals, supportive sneakers, or orthotics can all work to help support the plantar fascia. A good rule of thumb is if the arch feels relief when you are wearing the shoe, sneaker, or orthotic, it's probably doing its job. You don't have to get fancy with orthotics; research supports that in most cases, when attempting to relieve plantar fasciitis, an over-the-counter orthotic will work just as well as custom-made orthotics from a podiatrist. If you are still experiencing symptoms, however, we recommend seeking professional medical treatment.

If you are dealing with chronic plantar fasciitis, the treatment is often more aggressive. This is where calf stretching, foam rolling, trigger point therapy, soft tissue mobilization, and self-massage and myofascial release (see chapter 4) can be helpful.

Cuboid Syndrome

Cuboid syndrome is often self-diagnosed as plantar fasciitis. While of similar origins (both can stem from either a hyper- or hypomobile arch, acute trauma, or repetitive stress), these two injuries do have some key differences. Cuboid syndrome is the inflammation and possible dislocation of the cuboid bone, which is located on the outside of your foot, or of the peroneal longus tendon, which passes through the cuboid bone before wrapping underneath your foot to help make up your arch.

While cuboid syndrome and plantar fasciitis are different injuries, similar treatments apply. First you need to diagnose if the arch is hypo- or hypermobile and then follow the recommended rehab exercises. For the cuboid bone and the lateral peroneals, foam rolling and soft tissue work can loosen up the muscles that attach to and mobilize the bone. This region of the foot often gets locked up, causing uneven load distribution. Sometimes, cuboid syndrome requires a special manipulation, known as the cuboid whip, from a physical therapist or chiropractor. This procedure can help to realign the bone and promote healthy joint kinematics. If you are receiving treatment from one of these professionals, they will tell you if this manipulation is right for you.

Night Splints

A common question we are asked, and one that you might have come across via Dr. Google, is whether a night splint is appropriate for you. This is a tough question. A night splint may help some patients alleviate symptoms, but it's not a one-size-fits-all solution.

Try to pay attention to the resting position of your foot throughout the day and especially at night. Do you find yourself constantly pointing your toes, or does your foot seem to naturally gravitate toward a more plantar flexed and inverted position (which puts your Achilles in a shortened position)? Do you sleep with your feet in plantar flexion (say, on your belly with your legs outstretched, so your feet are facing downward)? Like anything, too much of any one position can be counterproductive, so using tools to help your feet spend time in another position can be helpful.

If your feet stay pretty consistently in one position or the other and you're dealing with plantar fasciitis or Achilles tendinitis, a night splint might be worth a try. It may have varying degrees of efficacy, but the night splint is not going to hurt anything. If it doesn't feel helpful, stop using it. Furthermore, you don't necessarily have to wear it throughout the whole night; even a few hours can achieve results.

Training Considerations

When dealing with plantar fasciitis during a training cycle, runners often ask, "Is this something that I can run through?" While plantar fasciitis alone is not necessarily a sidelining injury, there are several things to consider. A big one is compensation. Dr. Aguillard herself has gotten a stress fracture in the little toe bones on the outer side of her foot due to a compensatory running stride that she developed from running through plantar fasciitis. We generally discourage runners experiencing plantar fasciitis from doing speed work and encourage them to try to run every other day until symptoms begin to improve. Depending on how severe the injury is, a substantial break from running may be necessary.

Conclusion

While the material covered in this chapter is useful as a first line of defense when dealing with plantar fasciitis, it is essential to get to the root of the problem. Seeking help from a professional can be a game changer, especially for plantar fasciitis, which can easily become a chronic problem and cause compensation while running—which will lead to even more problems!

CHAPTER 11

Achilles Tendinitis

The Achilles tendon is the strongest tendon in the body. It is what gives humans the ability to walk, jump, and run. In fact, the Achilles tendon is a key structure that separates us from our primate cousins, and it makes us more efficient at covering longer distances than many other animals . . . including horses!

However, because it's so integral to our running stride, it's impossible to run without placing a good deal of stress on this tendon. To be fair, it's built to receive stress; the Achilles tendon can absorb ground forces of up to eight times our body weight, and it does so in order to efficiently transfer that energy and propel us forward. As a result, however, it is one of the most commonly injured structures on runners' bodies.

Let's start by finding the Achilles tendon on the body. If you find your calf muscle and follow it down your leg, you'll notice that it starts to narrow as it approaches the heel bone. This is your Achilles tendon (figure 11.1).

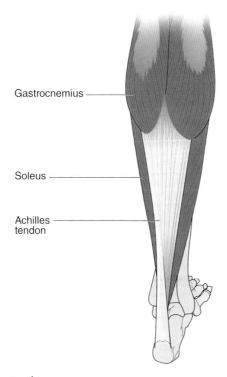

Gastrocnemius

Soleus

Achilles tendon

Figure 11.1 Achilles tendon.

Causes of Achilles Tendinitis

One common cause of Achilles tendinitis—and many other running injuries, as you'll see—is doing too much too soon. Tissue adaptation occurs slowly over time by increasing the load or stress that is applied to it (miles run per week or intensity of workouts are examples of running loads or stresses). Ramping up your running intensity or mileage too quickly doesn't give your tissues—in this case, the Achilles tendon—time to adapt to the increased demand of running. This is when injury can occur.

Another cause has less to do with the Achilles tendon itself than with the structure that surrounds it. It's a specific type of connective tissue sheath, or case, called a *peritenon*. The purpose of the peritenon is to keep the Achilles tendon lubricated so that it can smoothly transition the forces it is receiving. If the peritenon surrounding the Achilles tendon becomes stiff or restricted, inflammation and injury can occur. In fact, what we typically label *Achilles tendinitis* is often injury or inflammation of the peritenon that surrounds the Achilles. Restriction in the peritenon—and the resulting Achilles tendinitis—can come from stiffness in the ankles, arches, or plantar fascia. It can also be caused by tightness in the calf muscles, or by overworking your calves due to deficiencies or compensations in your running gait.

Diagnosis

An Achilles tendinitis diagnosis is straightforward on the surface: Any pain, inflammation, or discomfort on or around the structure is commonly diagnosed as Achilles tendinitis (figure 11.2).

Early stages of Achilles tendinitis may cause symptoms only during running or jumping, but the tendinitis can progress to the point at which symptoms arise from pushing up on your toes, going up and down stairs, or even walking on flat surfaces. Often, symptoms decrease as your body gets

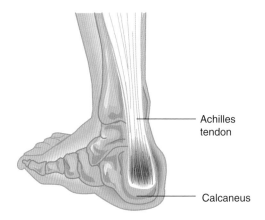

Achilles
tendon

Calcaneus

Figure 11.2   Common site of Achilles tendon inflammation.

moving and the tissue warms up, only to return when activity is stopped. This happens because, as your body starts to move and warm up, the calf muscles loosen, which takes some of the strain off the Achilles tendon and surrounding structures. Then, when you stop and your muscles tighten up again, the strain on the Achilles tendon returns.

Tendinitis Versus Tendinosis

Left untreated, Achilles tendinitis commonly progresses to Achilles *tendinosis*. However, distinguishing between these two injuries can get tricky. From a diagnosis standpoint, the easiest measure is time.

In a clinical setting—if, for example, you get evaluated by a physical therapist—you will be asked how long you've been experiencing symptoms. If the duration has been for less than six weeks, they will probably diagnose you with tendinitis. Tendinitis, as we have discussed, is the inflammation of the tendon, caused by microtears that happen due to acute overloading of the tendon by forces that are too heavy, too sudden, or too demanding. Over time, these microtears can cause more substantial tissue degeneration, as well as structural changes in the anatomy of the tendon or heel bone on which the tendon inserts, leading to tendinosis (Bass 2012). Therefore, if your symptoms have lasted longer than six weeks, you will probably be diagnosed with tendinosis.

As we described in chapter 6, tendinosis (figure 11.3) is the degeneration of the tendon's collagen in response to chronic overuse. What happens here is that instead of becoming inflamed as the result of overload, the tendon thickens and increases stiffness. Misaligned, immature collagen fibers start to build up—meaning that instead of providing strong, parallel alignment that facilitates strength with load bearing, the fibers are disorganized and not as structurally sound (Asplund and Best 2013).

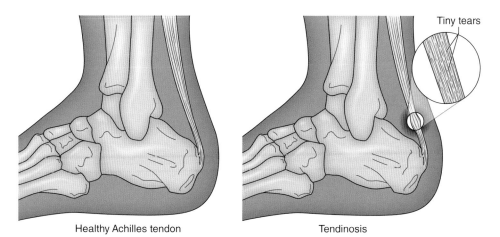

Healthy Achilles tendon   Tendinosis

Figure 11.3 Healthy Achilles tendon and Achilles tendinosis.

Case Study: Morgan

Morgan presents to physical therapy complaining of pain and swelling in the back of his lower leg, midway between his calf and his heel. Morgan reports he had taken time off from doing structured workouts for a while, and last week ran ten 200-meter hill sprints for the first time in quite some time. Morgan reports that during the activity, he felt totally fine, but when he got home he started to feel pain in the back of his foot.

Observation: Morgan has a slight limp when he walks, due to the pain he's feeling at the back of his heel.

Diagnosis: Achilles tendinitis.

Treatment: Treatment for Morgan consists of soft tissue mobilization and the Graston technique on his calf, arch, and Achilles tendon, performed by his physical therapist. He is instructed to wear a shoe with a lift for two weeks and do calf stretching while in the acute phase of injury rehabilitation. Once Morgan is able to walk without pain, treatment progresses to calf strengthening, plyometric loading, and posterior chain neuromuscular reeducation (getting the calf, hamstring, and glute to work together). Eccentric strengthening is limited until several weeks have passed, because Morgan's injury had a sudden onset (see page 131 for further discussion).

Tendon Rupture

Acute tendon rupture occurs most often during an explosive running or jumping motion. Although this type of injury is much more common in sports such as basketball, in rare cases it can also occur with running, particularly at faster speeds or on a tendon that's been chronically inflamed.

To avoid a big injury like this one, train smartly and maintain proper mobility and strength in the area surrounding your Achilles tendon. This is especially important after age 35, when degenerative changes that occur with age will start to put the Achilles tendon more at risk for a tear or rupture. The other time to be extra careful is when you've been diagnosed with tendinosis, because your tendon will be less structurally sound and, consequently, more prone to rupture or tear.

Treatment and Prevention of Achilles Tendinitis and Achilles Tendinosis

Treatment for Achilles injuries can differ depending on whether your Achilles injury falls into the tendinitis or tendinosis category. Although there is some overlap between treatment of the two injuries, understanding how they differ can increase the efficacy of healing.

Heel Lift

In the acute phases of Achilles tendinitis, when the tendon is swollen and inflamed, do as much as you can to protect the tendon from extra stress. This is when using a heel lift can come in handy. We often encourage patients to look for a shoe with a higher heel-toe profile (versus a more minimal or lower-profile shoe); this can make a big difference in the demand that's put on the tendon in both walking and running. Please note, however, that this is a temporary fix. Restricting movement may reduce pain and inflammation in a region but will not address the root of the problem, which is the inability of the tendon to handle load. Once the inflammation has calmed down, it's critical to reintroduce movement and loading through the Achilles to build resilience and prevent the injury from occurring again.

Stretch With Caution

While regular calf stretching can be a useful tool to prevent Achilles tendinitis from forming, in the acute phases of tendinitis, lengthening the calves can actually cause excessive strain, leading to further pain and inflammation. Gentle stretching is usually okay, but cranking the calf into a deep stretch will not cure your Achilles tendinitis and can often make things worse. For more information on how to effectively stretch your calf, see the 3D calf stretch in chapter 6. Night splints are occasionally prescribed for Achilles tendinitis. These are discussed in the sidebar on page 124 in chapter 10.

Self-Myofascial Release and Massage

While calf stretches should be done minimally and very gently, foam rolling or massaging the calves can help to decrease the strain that's being put on the Achilles and can be done a bit more aggressively (see chapter 6 for the technique). It's helpful for both tendinitis and tendinosis injuries, as well as preventing Achilles tendinitis from occurring at all.

We also recommend specifically mobilizing the Achilles tendon and peritenon to get the Achilles to glide back and forth in the sheath by freeing up restrictions there. Gentle massage along the tendon with your fingers can help to promote this type of mobility (figure 11.4). Sit on the floor with legs extended, toes pointed to the ceiling. Cross one leg over the other so you can reach the Achilles. You may also press a lacrosse ball right above the Achilles and work your way up little by little, incorporating ankle pumps up and down or circles with your foot for active release.

If you find this technique tricky to self-administer, a physical therapist with specific training in running-related injuries can be a good resource to help with stickier tendons.

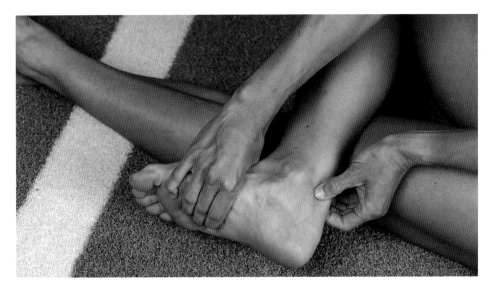

Figure 11.4   Self-massage of the Achilles.

Compression

Generally, compression helps to promote blood flow to the region that is being compressed, which speeds up the recovery process. Therefore, compression socks, sleeves, or boots can be very useful for managing both Achilles tendinitis and Achilles tendinosis. Plus, it's easy: You can wear compression socks after your run, around the house, underneath your normal clothes, and even to bed at night.

Currently, there is no evidence to support using compression during running to prevent or heal Achilles tendinitis. However, there is evidence to support using it while running to reduce pain in the area. This might sound like masking the symptoms, but it's actually a logical part of chronic injury management. Part of the issue with a chronic injury is that the brain becomes hypersensitive to discomfort in the region of the injury. In the case of Achilles tendinosis, for instance, the nerves surrounding the tendon become extra sensitive, which leads to increased perceived pain in the injured area. The key word here is *perceived*—your injury may not necessarily still be there, but your nerves are firing at the slightest prompt, so your body is "feeling" pain. Once the injury itself has been managed, particularly if it is chronic, you need to decrease your perceived pain awareness. Compression helps with this.

Eccentric Strengthening

If you've had chronic Achilles issues, you'll be familiar with eccentric calf strengthening, or the Alfredson protocol, which is considered to be the gold standard of treatment for Achilles tendinitis and Achilles tendinosis. Dr. Alfredson was an orthopedist who suffered from chronic Achilles pain. In an effort to rupture the tendon himself so that a colleague would perform surgery on him, he began to load the tendon as heavily as he could with eccentric muscle contraction of the calf (considered to be the strongest, most intense type of muscle contraction). To his surprise, rather than rupturing the tendon like he had intended, he found that his tendon healed.

Ever since Dr. Alfredson's discovery, repetitive eccentric loading of the Achilles tendon has been used successfully to treat Achilles tendinosis. Eccentric loading can be extremely helpful in promoting blood flow to a chronically injured area. This encourages the continued development of new collagen fibers, which in turn helps to restore alignment of these fibers for increased strength and resilience to loading forces.

However, if you are going to use an eccentric loading protocol for treatment, do it correctly and under the right conditions. If you are experiencing tendinitis or the tissue is acutely inflamed, *eccentric loading can make your symptoms worse*. Only when you are dealing with chronic symptoms without acute inflammation or swelling, or if you've been given approval by your doctor or physical therapist, should you implement an eccentric loading protocol.

It's recommended to perform eccentric calf loading (what many athletes dub a *calf raise*) double-legged in the beginning: up on two feet, down on two feet. The focus should be on a slow, controlled descent (figure 11.5*a*). While the research says to do as many repetitions as possible, 10 to 30 reps is sufficient. If you can tolerate 30 reps pain-free, with no uptick in symptoms within 24 to 48 hours of completion, you can progress to up on two feet, down on one foot (figure 11.5*b*). Then, when this routine becomes tolerable and fails to provoke any symptoms, the next progression would be up on two feet, down on two feet with the backs of your feet hanging off of a step or incline so that your heels drop past a neutral position; this does a good job of stretching the tendon and, when done repeatedly, can help to realign the distorted collagen fibers (figure 11.5*c*). The final step would be to go up on two feet, down on one foot with your heel hanging off a step (figure 11.5*d*).

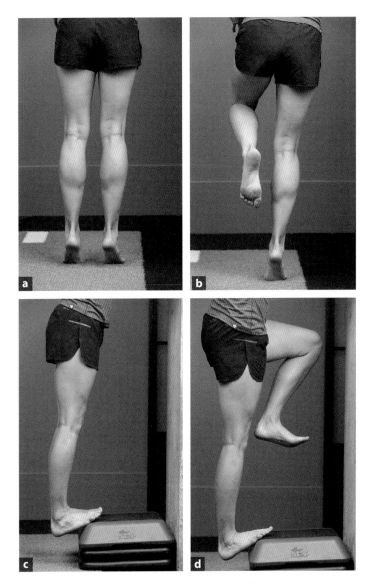

Figure 11.5   Alfredson protocol: *(a)* double-legged to neutral; *(b)* single-legged to neutral; *(c)* double-legged past neutral; *(d)* single-legged past neutral.

Case Study: Taylor

Taylor presents to physical therapy complaining of heel pain that has been persistent for the past few months. Taylor reports that his heel has felt "off" for a while, and he's struggled with heel pain off and on for as long as he can remember. In the last few weeks, things seemed to have taken a turn for the worse, and Taylor is worried he's going to start to compensate his running form.

Observation: Taylor's Achilles tendon is thicker than normal, and he has pain at the base of the heel, where the Achilles tendon is inserting into the bone.

Diagnosis: Tendinosis.

Treatment: Taylor's treatment begins with a manual approach similar to Morgan's treatment: calf, Achilles, and plantar fascia mobilization plus ankle joint manipulations to restore full range of motion. Taylor is also started on the Alfredson protocol of eccentric contractions because his injury is already in a chronic state. Once Taylor demonstrates full range of motion, pain-free walking, and tolerance to single-leg eccentric loading past the neutral position (i.e., starting and ending with the heel off a step), he is cleared to return to easy running and begin plyometric training. (Adding plyometric training to tendon rehab increases the buffer zone of forces the structure can handle, beyond running, without pain, so it's less likely to fatigue when running.)

Training Considerations

Much like plantar fasciitis, a runner can continue to run and train through mild cases of Achilles tendinitis and tendinosis when proper modifications are made. Here are a few elements to keep in mind if you are continuing to run with Achilles pain:

- *Form:* If you are not properly engaging your glutes with each push-off, your calves—and, by extension, Achilles tendons—are being placed under considerable stress as you attempt forward propulsion. This can stem from weakness in the glutes or tightness in the hip flexors that limits hip extension. While we encourage you to have a physical therapist evaluate your form, a telltale sign of not engaging the glutes is soreness in your calves and quads after a hard run or workout. See chapters 7 and 8 for exercises to improve glute activation and hip mobility.

- *Footwear:* Choosing a shoe with a higher profile (i.e., heel-toe drop) can reduce the workload of your Achilles tendon and decrease stress on this region. Remember, this is only a temporary fix, not a cure.

- *Surface:* A smooth, flat surface decreases the work required of the calf and is preferable to hillier terrain, grass, dirt, or trails, which will be more demanding on the Achilles tendon.

• *Pacing:* See if you can find the sweet spot, a comfortable pace that is not too fast and not too slow. Higher-intensity running puts much more force, or load, on the tendon and should be avoided, but running significantly slower than your natural cadence can also put increased demand on the Achilles tendon, due to the shorter stride length.

Conclusion

Whether or not you are choosing to run through your Achilles injury, remember: This book does not replace checking in with your doctor, podiatrist, or physical therapist to get to the root of your injury. Tendon injuries are some of the most complex and finicky ones out there, and the Achilles tendon is no exception. So try your best to be patient as you work through diagnosing and treating your pain. With patience and persistence, you can get through this!

CHAPTER 12
Shin Splints

You might have experienced shin splints, or medial tibial stress syndrome, when you first started running—they're arguably the most common injury to plague novice runners (Thacker et al. 2002). The same goes for runners who are getting back into running after extended time off: Your shins can often be the first part of your body to get sore. In this chapter, we dig into the why and how behind these tendencies.

Causes of Shin Splints

Running involves high-impact repetitive loading forces that place stress on your entire body. Since your foot, followed by your tibia, are the first parts of your body to strike the ground, your foot and tibia absorb the most impact forces each time you land. It's these stresses, repeated with every foot strike, that cause tiny microtears in your muscles and microfractures in your bones. If enough of these microtears and microfractures occur without sufficient recovery, inflammation accumulates, and boom—it's as if someone stuck a splinter inside your shin! That's the origin of the shorthand name *shin splints*.

It's because of their tendency to underrecover that novice runners often suffer from shin splints, regardless of biomechanics, build, strength, or running form. Therefore, the first line of defense, and often the simplest fix, is having a proper training plan that prevents you from ramping up your intensity or mileage too quickly. (We share more about developing such a plan in chapter 15.) If you do start to experience some discomfort on the inside of your shin, you don't necessarily need to stop running, but you do need to address it. Continuing to push through shin pain can lead to the development of a stress fracture, which *will* stop you from running.

Training errors are not the only actions that can lead to shin splints, however. Other factors that can increase your risk include overpronation or the type of surface you are running on (Thacker et al. 2002). And then there are form or biomechanical errors. Two of the most common biomechanical errors are overstriding and overworking the calves, so we're going to address those here. That said, there are many other biomechanical factors that can lead to shin splints, so seeking an evaluation from a physical therapist is your best bet to get a recovery plan that is customized for you.

Overstriding

Overstriding (figure 12.1*a*), or having a stride length that is too long, causes your foot to land in front of your body instead of under your body. We discuss foot placement in greater detail in chapter 16, but the primary reason you want your foot to land under your body (figure 12.1*b*), specifically your pelvis, is that it enables your body to more evenly distribute the impact of the landing across your joints and better absorb the impact of your landing using muscles in your hips. On the other hand, when your foot lands too far in front of your body, it causes your shinbone and leg to absorb too much of that force—which, over time, is what will lead to injury.

Overstriding can happen despite the type of foot strike a runner has (heel, mid-, or forefoot). We've seen a number of forefoot strikers who still overstride, which contributes to both overworking the calf muscle and less-than-ideal shock absorption. However, the combination of overstriding with a hefty heel strike is a sure recipe for shin splints—there is simply too much force going straight through the foot and into the tibia. An athlete with this type of running form may also experience problems further up the chain, such as knee pain, hip pain, or low back pain.

Calf Overuse

Another biomechanical error that can contribute to shin splints is having very tight (i.e., overworked) calves—often due to tight hips and a lack of glute–hamstring engagement. (For folks who spend most of their day sitting

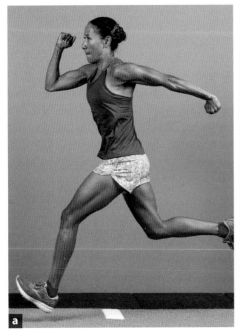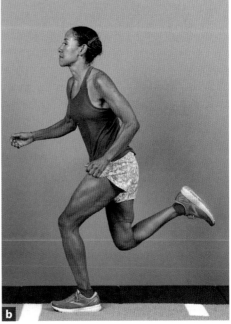

Figure 12.1 Runner *(a)* overstriding and *(b)* with proper stride length.

in front of a computer, we refer to this latter issue as *sleepy butt syndrome*.) Because the muscles up the chain are not firing properly, the runner is dependent on the calf for push-off.

If your calves are too tight from being overworked, this may lead to decreased dorsiflexion of the ankle joint (the ability of the ankle to bend so the shin bone moves past the toes) in landing, which limits the ability of the foot to load and absorb shock. If the ankle is limited in dorsiflexion, a common compensation is increasing pronation, which researchers have linked to shin splints (Moen et al. 2009). One other biomechanical factor that contributes to shin splints is increased speed of loading, or a tight calf overpowering the eccentric strength of the anterior tibia. In simpler terms, this means that the calf is so strong at propelling you forward that the muscles that help with shock absorption can't keep up with the rate at which you're moving, leading to painful inflammation in the shin area.

In summary, tight or overworked calves can cause a number of mobility limitations throughout the foot and ankle that, in turn, can cause compensations in running stride. These compensations then lead to increased forces on the shin, causing inflammation of the muscles that attach to the tibia, and there you have it: shin splints.

Diagnosis

Despite how common shin splints are, most people aren't quite sure *what* they are. Even in the medical community, there is some debate on how to properly define a shin splint. In this book, we are referring to a shin splint as inflammation of the muscles, tendons, and bones that comprise the inside of the shin. A shin splint is not a stress reaction or fracture of the tibia (shinbone). It's more superficial than a bone stress injury, in which the injury has progressed to the point of weakening the integrity of the bone.

With a traditional shin splint, the athlete feels the pain along the inside of the tibia. This is why, if you were to look at your medical chart when receiving treatment for a shin splint, you'd probably see a diagnosis of *medial tibial stress syndrome*.

Red Flags: When It's Not Actually a Shin Splint

Most runners cringe when they hear the word stress fracture—it's commonly understood that this can mean months on the sidelines. Shin splints are a straightforward signal from your body that you might be heading down stress fracture road if something doesn't change. And in fact, you need to make sure what you're calling a shin splint isn't already a stress fracture.

One way to distinguish a shin splint from a stress fracture or stress reaction is how it feels on a run: Shin splints will typically feel better as a run progresses, while the more serious bone injury often presents as a consistent, dull ache that stays the same or gets slightly worse during or after a run. Shin splints can often be alleviated with a few days of rest or training modifications, and they typically (although not always) affect a broader area of the shinbone. With stress fractures, the pain is usually more localized and can cause discomfort with walking or even just carrying something heavy, like groceries. Continuing to run on a stress fracture can lead to a full-blown break of the bone and, in the worst-case scenario, surgery. So if you're feeling uncertain about the root of your shin pain, definitely see a medical professional.

Another serious medical condition that can sometimes present as a shin splint is compartment syndrome, or localized pressure in certain muscles of the body. One of the most common areas this affects is your lower legs. It can present as a tightness, cramping, swelling, or discomfort of the muscles around the tibia or shinbone, and if left untreated, can start to affect the nerves in this region and lead to numbness, weakness, or, in extreme cases, temporary paralysis of your lower leg. If you think you are experiencing signs of compartment syndrome, seek immediate treatment from a health care professional.

Case Study: Ava

Ava is training for her first 5K and started having pain in her shins. She presents to physical therapy saying that she has pain in her shins at the beginning of every run. As she warms up, the pain seems to go away, but she's left with some residual soreness after she runs.

Observation: Ava has foot pronation and limited ankle dorsiflexion, along with increased tension in the relaxed muscle of both calves.

Diagnosis: Shin splints (medial tibial stress syndrome).

Treatment: Ava's physical therapist performs manual therapy to release tension in her calves, assigns her anterior tibial strengthening (ankle dorsiflexion) exercises, and provides her with form cues to help her regulate her cadence when she gets back to running. The therapist also educates her on how to construct a proper training plan and progression (see chapter 15).

Treatment and Prevention of Shin Splints

Now that we've explained what a shin splint is and how you could have developed this injury, let's take a deeper dive into how to manage shin splints and prevent them from happening. Often by modifying a few factors within your training, you can reduce the pain in your shin without having to sit on the sideline completely. We know the last thing most runners want to hear is "just take some time off."

Training

Since the most common cause of shin splints is training error, let's talk about a few common mistakes. First, track your mileage (or "time on feet"), and ensure that you are not ramping up your running too quickly. Limiting additions to your weekly mileage can be a great first line of defense to reduce the severity of your shin splints and avoid having to take time off from running—and also to prevent shin splints from occurring in the first place.

Working with an experienced running coach can help you to avoid this all-too-common mistake, but you can put together a smart plan yourself, too. A 10 percent increase per week in overall mileage is a good guideline, but it's not the answer for every runner. If you're starting from the couch, begin by running no more than every other day, and if you have a history of bone injuries or shin splints, running only every third day will give your body the time it needs to adjust to the training. (For more training tips, see chapter 15.)

Another factor to consider is surface. If you are doing a lot of your running on a sidewalk or concrete surface, this could be contributing to your shin pain. By choosing a softer surface, you can decrease the amount of force being applied to your shin and can often continue running with less pain, rather than sitting out completely. Dirt trails are great, but if you don't have access, there are other solutions. As boring as it may seem, jogging around a soccer field will allow you to safely increase your mileage while lessening the amount of force that's loading through your body. Plus, the variable surface of grass actually causes the muscles of your foot and ankle to work harder, which can help your body become more resilient to injury. A local track is another great option, because the rubber surface is more forgiving than concrete. Treadmills also fall into the category of softer surface, but be careful. Treadmill running has also been linked to an increase in overstriding (a natural compensation when running on a surface that is moving toward you), and overstriding can contribute to developing shin splints.

Biomechanics

Although it can be harder to adjust biomechanics than to adjust weekly mileage or running surfaces, understanding the biomechanics that can contribute to excessive loading through the shin and making adjustments to your running form can also play a pivotal role in preventing or eradicating shin splints.

Overstriding

As discussed earlier, overstriding directly results in more impact force being absorbed by your shin. If your foot is landing in front of you, rather than the force of the ground being transmitted up the leg, the brunt of the force goes into your shin and then your knee. If the issue that caused your shin splint turns out to be overstriding, there are several running drills that can help you to increase turnover and improve where your foot lands relative to your body's center of mass. (This means they work well to prevent shin splints, too!) The progression of high knee drills and butt kicks described in chapter 16 will improve your ability to land beneath your own center of gravity.

One drill to add to the mix is the claw (figure 12.2).

Paying attention to your cadence can also help to reduce overstriding. An optimal cadence is around 180 steps per minute, but even just a 5 to 10 percent increase from whatever your current cadence is can make a huge difference. Alter your cadence by focusing on taking shorter, quicker steps. A smartphone metronome app or a jogging tunes app can help you coordinate your footfall with a higher cadence, thereby reducing the impact on your shins.

Lastly, because changing your form is very hard and takes a lot of time, strengthening the muscles in the front of your shin in the meantime can help build resilience in the tissue, helping it better handle the force of the ground. The heel walk on page 141 will help, as will the 3D banded strength exercises in chapter 6.

The Claw

Face a wall and put both palms against the wall for balance. Stand on one foot. Raise the knee of your working leg until your thigh is parallel to the ground (figure 12.2*a*). Cycle your leg down toward the ground and scrape back (figure 12.2*b*), as though pushing the ground behind you, before flexing your knee and bringing your leg back up. The goal is for the foot to strike the ground underneath your body instead of landing in front of you. Repeat 10 to 15 times per leg.

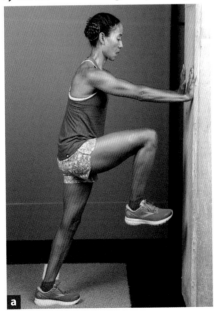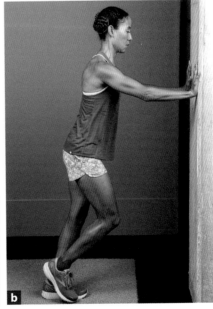

Figure 12.2   Claw: *(a)* starting position; *(b)* cycle the leg down, and push back.

Heel Walk

Lift all ten toes up off ground so you are walking on your heels (figure 12.3). Focus on controlling ankle dorsiflexion as you walk around a room.

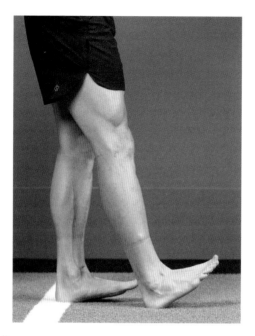

Figure 12.3   Heel walk.

Calf Overuse

If you find that your shin splints are caused by tight or overworked calves, there are a series of things you can do:

- Stretch your hip flexors. See the 3D kneeling hip flexor stretch described in chapter 7.
- Activate your glutes functionally by using the claw exercise described earlier in this chapter and B-skips described in chapter 16.
- Foam roll and stretch those calves. It's going to take time for stretches and activation exercises to work their magic. In the short term, if you continue to run, your calves are still going to be working too hard. Give them this little extra bit of TLC. They'll thank you.
- Strengthen your anterior shins. Exercises to help this include heel walks and the 3D banded strength exercises in chapter 6.

- Use compression. Slipping on a pair of compression socks after a run will promote increased circulation to the shins and calves, which can help to speed up recovery and reduce inflammation. If you have access, the Voodoo Band and Normatec Compression boots are an even more intense way to include compression in your postrun routine.

- Try running with form cues. It's one thing to stretch and activate; it's another thing to put it into practice while running. For instance, all the glute activation in the world will do you no good if you can't engage your glutes as a part of your stride. One way to do this is to think about pushing the ground back and away from you while you run. Still not working? Try leaning forward a bit more than seems natural, to put the glute in a biomechanically advantageous position. Finally, as opposed to increasing the work other muscles are doing, try to decrease the work your calves are doing by focusing on keeping your feet relaxed and "floppy."

Conclusion

While they are common, shin splints are not the most complicated running injury. Even just understanding and staying aware of the interplay between training and running mechanics can make a huge difference when it comes to avoiding this classic overuse injury. Train smartly and give your calves some TLC, and you'll leave shin splints in the dust.

CHAPTER 13

Hamstring Tendinitis and Tendinopathy

The first thing that comes to mind when we think of hamstring injury in runners is the dreaded "pop"—the sudden and acute tear of a muscle often associated with sprinting, jumping, or another high-power motion. Yet hamstring injuries come in all shapes and sizes, from acute "pop" injuries to chronic tendinosis that plagues the muscle where it attaches to the bone. In this chapter, we will break down injuries that can occur in these powerful muscles and talk about strategies that can help prevent and heal them.

The hamstring is composed of three different muscles: biceps femoris, semitendinosus, and semimembranosus (figure 13.1). All three muscles are innervated by branches of the sciatic nerve, and all three originate from the ischial tuberosity (also known as the *sit bone*). These muscles attach behind the knee, crossing both the hip joint and the knee joint. These are powerful muscles that play a role in both movement and stabilization at two joints: the hip and the knee.

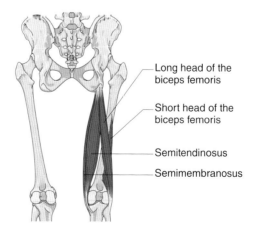

Long head of the biceps femoris

Short head of the biceps femoris

Semitendinosus

Semimembranosus

Figure 13.1 Hamstrings.

While similar in origin, the three muscles' distinct insertion points are important to understand for correctly diagnosing and treating hamstring injury. The *biceps femoris* muscle attaches to the fibula and the outside of the tibia (the bones that make up your lower leg). If you're experiencing lateral knee pain, the biceps femoris can sometimes be the culprit. The *semitendinosus* muscle attaches to the inside of the knee, or the pes anserine, a common insertion point of the gracilis adductor, hamstring, and sartorius hip flexor. Any excess tension or friction here can lead to bursitis or inflammation of this common insertion point. Finally, the *semimembranosus* muscle attaches to the medial tibial condyle, close to the meniscus, which is inside the knee joint. Pain or tightness here can be closely linked with medial meniscus pain.

Hamstring Function in Running

Before we go further down the injury path, let's discuss what the hamstring is supposed to do while you're running. Anatomically, the hamstring muscles are designed to extend the hip and flex or bend the knee, which means they're critical to maintaining control throughout the running gait cycle. Let's break it down.

Push-Off

Along with the glutes, the hamstrings are major players in force production during the push-off phase of the running stride. This means they help to convert the ground reaction force (the force of your body hitting the ground) into kinetic energy that propels you forward by extending the hip and then the knee. Weakness or underfunctioning in the glutes can lead to overworking the hamstrings—which can, in turn, lead to injury—so in strength and plyometric training, it's important to strengthen these muscle groups together and include specific exercises that target the glutes.

Swing Phase

The hamstrings are the main muscle group that controls the swing phase by decelerating the forward movement of the hip and knee, or anterior pelvic tilt. This is when the most force is going through the hamstrings eccentrically and when the muscle is most at risk for injury. Overstriding can put more force through the muscle at this stage of gait because you are demanding more force from the hamstrings while they are firing from an overlengthened position. Therefore, actively think about pulling your leg back to the ground as you are striding forward, rather than reaching with it. (More on this in chapter 16.)

Ground Contact

When you're transitioning from the swing phase to making contact with the ground, the hamstrings must actively work to pull the leg back to the ground. Once again, overstriding can cause injury in this phase of the running stride, as well; it forces the hip to move through a greater degree of relative extension so the hamstrings must work harder to pull the foot back underneath the knee at impact.

Stabilization

Stabilization is an often overlooked—but critical—role of the hamstrings during running. When the foot hits the ground, all the muscles around the knee (quads, hamstrings, adductors, and calf) must synergistically contract to stabilize the knee. This collective contraction does two things. First, it allows for maximum use of the energy that has been stored at impact in the Achilles tendon, increasing running economy. Second, it protects the knee from taking the full brunt of the ground force impact, thus protecting it from injury. At the same time as they're contracting to protect the knee and gather propulsive force, the hamstrings are also stabilizing and preventing too much anterior movement of the pelvis, helping to maintain neutrality in both the hip and spine (Beer 2019).

Hamstring Tightness

It seems to be common knowledge that runners have tight hamstrings. We want to break this down a little bit, however, because "tight" hamstrings are often not quite what you think they are. In standing, walking, and running, the hamstrings (along with your core) play a critical role in holding the pelvis in a neutral position, meaning the hamstrings counter the forces that pull the pelvis forward into an anterior pelvic tilt (figure 13.2*a* and figure 13.2*b*). These forces can be caused by tightness in your hip flexors, which pulls the pelvis forward, or they can arise from overstretched, weak hamstrings failing to provide adequate support and stability (Beatty et al. 2017).

   A common mistake that many runners make to help ease or prevent hamstring injury is to overstretch the hamstrings. There's a reason most runners have tight hamstrings, and it's also why you typically don't see ballet dancers—who have excellent hamstring mobility—winning races. Generally, a tight hamstring is a strong hamstring. Therefore, as a runner, it's actually okay to have tight hamstrings! We just don't want your hamstrings so tight that they pop, which is the reason to do appropriate soft tissue maintenance. However, sometimes this feeling of tightness can come from hamstrings that are functioning in a chronically overlengthened state, meaning that the hamstrings are not adequately stabilizing the pelvis.

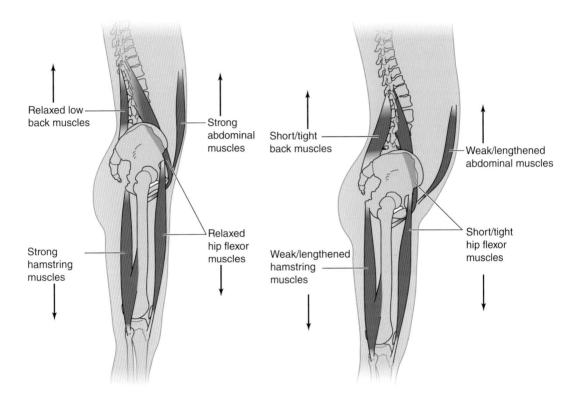

Figure 13.2   *(a)* Neutral pelvis, versus *(b)* anteriorly rotated pelvis.

If this is the case, it's common for your hamstrings to *feel* very tight. Think of the hamstring muscle like a rubber band that is stretched too far. If it's being pulled from one of its attachment sites, or functioning in a suboptimal position, you will perceive your hamstrings as being too tight, even though the hamstring is actually overlengthened.

To determine if your hamstrings might be overlengthened answer this simple question: Can you touch your toes? If you have no problem touching your toes, you are definitely not suffering from hamstring muscle tightness. In this case, you will benefit more from strengthening and stabilization exercises for the hamstrings and glutes than from working on stretching and increasing mobility. Yet when strengthening the hamstrings, it's critical to do so from a neutral position versus an overlengthened position. We do *not* want to be trying to generate a large force from a muscle in an overlengthened position—this is a recipe for disaster! If you are unable to touch your toes, we recommend working on hamstring mobility. However, there are many ways to do this, not all of which involve stretching.

Although stretching your hamstrings might give you that "hurts so good" feeling, any relief you feel comes mostly from the neuromuscular input that the stretch provides—that is, stretching sends a signal to your brain to relax taut muscle fibers. But be careful, because it only takes a gentle stimulus for this to occur. Overstretching the hamstrings, or putting force through the muscle under a lengthened position, can cause tearing, irritation, inflammation, weakness, or injury of the hamstring tendon. If you continue to put force through the injured muscle, even via stretching, your injury will only worsen (Beatty et al. 2017).

If you are a runner with overly tight hamstrings (you are unable to touch your toes), we recommend foam rolling and lacrosse ball trigger point work to try and improve soft tissue mobility and extensibility. Additionally, gentle stretching is okay, but try not to stretch the muscle beyond 90 degrees of hip flexion. For example, putting your leg up on a fence at or above your waist height while standing would be excessive. Try to keep the leg you are stretching closer to the height of your other knee.

Hamstring Trigger Point Release

Similar to the other foam rolling and self-massage myofascial release techniques we have discussed, using a lacrosse ball (or something similar) on the hamstrings is a very effective way to loosen up and mobilize the muscle belly (figure 13.3). We recommend being conservative around the site of most pain or injury, but digging fairly aggressively into the surrounding tissue. To perform the exercise, sit in a chair with the lacrosse ball underneath your leg. Similar to rolling the quads, start right above your knee and work your way up toward your glutes, pausing if you feel a spot that is knotty, tender, or hot—at those points, stop and bend your leg up and down or rock side to side for an active release. Try working the ball up and down three strips of hamstring: one up the middle between the two hamstring muscle bellies, one laterally focused on separating the hamstring from the IT band, and one medially near the hamstring–adductor junction. (Another player in hamstring dysfunction is the hamstring adhering, or becoming fascially stuck, to the adductors.)

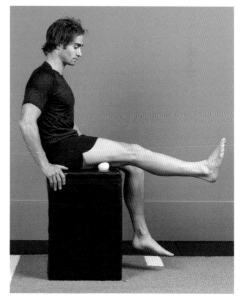

Figure 13.3 Trigger point release using a lacrosse ball.

Nerve Floss

If you are feeling any radiating pain (starting up in the hip and shooting down the leg) or have dealt with sciatica in the past, nerve glides or neural mobilization techniques are another useful tool in the toolbox. Rather than stretching the muscle, the goal is to mobilize the sciatic nerve as it runs through the hamstring muscle belly. Start by lying on your back and bending the knee of the affected leg toward your body, wrapping your arms around your thigh (figure 13.4a). Next, try to straighten your leg as much as you can by extending your knee (your foot should move toward the ceiling; figure 13.4b). Once the leg is extended as far as it will go, pull your toes toward your face (dorsiflexion; figure 13.4c). You should feel a stretch up the back of your leg. Next, relax your foot back into plantar flexion, and then lower your knee back down. Repeat in this order no more than 10 or 15 times; more than that can irritate the area.

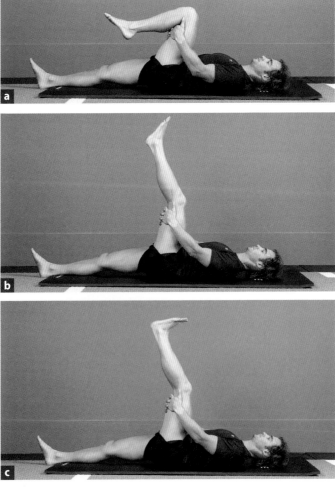

Figure 13.4   Nerve floss: *(a)* start position; *(b)* extend the leg; *(c)* flex the foot.

Diagnosis

Now that we understand the makeup and function of the hamstrings, let's delve into the ways they can be injured. Hamstring injuries can be divided into two basic types: acute or chronic. While the immediate injury can be one or the other, these two types of injury can also work in concert: Acute strain can lead to tendinitis, or tendinopathy can weaken the hamstring tendon and consequently lead to an acute injury.

Acute Injury

An acute hamstring injury involves tearing the muscle. If you are running and doing strides, a sprint, or hill surges and experience a sudden pop, pull, or jolt, please stop running and go back to chapter 3. Generally, heat application is recommended over ice. And absolutely do not stretch your hamstring! Gentle foam rolling is okay, but even minimal stretching can make an existing strain worse.

Chronic Injury: Hamstring Tendinitis and Tendinopathy

Chronic hamstring injury occurs more gradually and can be identified as a deeper discomfort in the back of the hip, butt, or less commonly, behind the knee. It can be hard to isolate specifically where the pain is coming from, and sometimes hamstring tendinitis can display similar symptoms to piriformis syndrome or sciatica. You might notice the pain increasing when running uphill, accelerating, opening up your stride, or running more quickly, but it will often feel fine on flat ground or when running slowly with shorter steps.

A good way to test for hamstring tendinopathy is through resistant knee flexion or hip extension. To test for this, you will need a partner to apply manual resistance to your leg. Lie on your abdomen on a table and bend your knee to 90 degrees. Have your partner apply a strong force, trying to push your knee back down (into knee extension) as you resist their force to the best of your ability (figure 13.5*a*). (Your partner should try to elicit a max contraction from you, but stop if you start to experience pain or symptoms.) Next, straighten your knee and lift your entire leg off the table, being careful not to overextend or lift from your low back. Your partner can apply the same resistive force, pushing your leg (we recommend a longer lever, applying the force closer to your ankle) toward the table (figure 13.5*b*). If either of these tests recreates your symptoms or causes pain or discomfort, your hamstring is probably the culprit. If both movements cause pain, you probably have proximal hamstring tendinitis or tendinopathy, but if only resisted knee flexion (not hip extension) causes pain, it's probably distal hamstring tendinopathy.

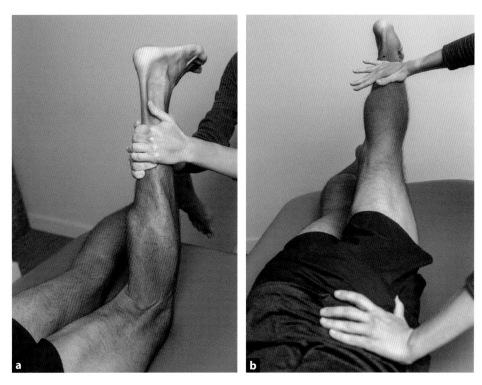

Figure 13.5 Resistant knee flexion and hip extension: *(a)* knee flexion; *(b)* hip extension.

Red Flags

When dealing with a hamstring injury, it's necessary to first rule out anything more serious that could be causing the pain—for instance a femoral or pelvic stress fracture, lumbosacral referral (meaning an injury to the low back and spinal cord that is "referring" pain to the hamstring), or hip pathology. See a medical professional if you aren't sure of the source of your pain.

The hamstring muscle group also runs closely alongside the sciatic nerve, which is the motor nerve to the hamstring muscles. The sciatic nerve can also contribute to pain in this region. Hamstring injury and sciatic nerve pain are not mutually exclusive; an irritated hamstring can compress the sciatic nerve, causing nerve pain or radiating pain, symptoms that are classically labeled *sciatica*. If you are experiencing symptoms consistent with sciatica, you could expect to see some improvements from hamstring rehabilitation.

Case Study: Ana

Ana reports that she has had left hamstring issues for a long time, but during her track workout yesterday, she felt a sharp pain and a pull in her hamstring, and now it hurts when she walks and is especially bad when she sits.

Observation: Ana presents with an anteriorly oriented pelvis that she maintains when standing, walking, and running. Her hamstring strength is sufficient, but her glutes also test weak. If you look at her muscular tone and definition, it's easy to see the muscle hypertrophy that exists in her hamstrings relative to her glutes. This is consistent with the chronic hamstring pain that she complains of. Ana is overly dependent on her hamstring muscles in her running gait (glute weakness) and is using them in a suboptimal position, which places increased torque on the muscle and tendon. On gait analysis, Ana overstrides, landing with her foot out in front of her body instead of underneath. This explains why speed work on the track could provoke her hamstring.

Diagnosis: Hamstring strain and hamstring tendinosis. (This is an example of how tendinotic hamstrings are more likely to pull, because they are less structurally sound.)

Treatment: Because of the acute onset of Ana's injury, treatment first consists of a series of hamstring isometric contractions, with an emphasis on pelvic orientation and engaging the hamstrings from a neutral pelvic position. Once she can tolerate it, Ana progresses to loading the hamstring while standing and working on strengthening the muscle dynamically, through concentric and eccentric loading. An emphasis is placed on co-contraction of the hamstring and glute muscles during strengthening exercises. Finally, Ana is able to progress to plyometric training and form drills. Ana's coach teaches her to pull her foot underneath her during her stride, increase her cadence, and lean forward to reduce the loading force on the hamstring with each step. Ana also has begun regularly incorporating deadlifts, hip thrusts, and single-leg Romanian deadlifts into her strength routine. Ana is back to training at a high level, pain-free.

Treatment and Prevention

An acutely injured runner should be able to tolerate their current exercises before progressing to the next phase. Make sure that the injured area is stressed enough to facilitate healing but isn't stressed so much that it stays inflamed and irritated. With both acute and chronic hamstring injury, you'll want to start with isometric hamstring strengthening and progress to concentric and then eccentric contractions. Likewise, start with a shorter lever arm (knee is bent closer to the butt), and then progress to a longer lever arm (performing exercises with knee in extension).

Isometric Hamstring Strengthening

The first step of rehabilitating a hamstring injury is to engage the hamstring muscle isometrically. In other words, you want to try to engage the muscle without changing the length or moving the bones. This activates the entire muscle and tendon, increasing recruitment of the muscle fibers and blood flow to the tendon without shortening or lengthening the muscle. The isometric bridge is an exercise that does just that.

Isometric Bridge

Lie on your back and create a bridge with your hips by digging your heels into the ground (figure 13.6a); you should feel the hamstring muscles turn on. Try holding the bridge for 30 to 60 seconds. If you sit at a desk for most of the day, you can also do this while in a seated position (figure 13.6b). Aim to activate the muscle once an hour, eight times a day.

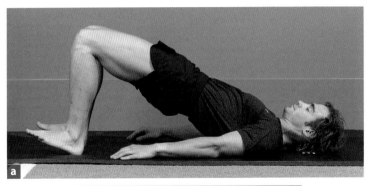

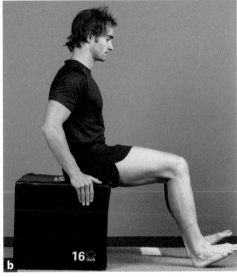

Figure 13.6   *(a)* Isometric bridge and *(b)* seated hamstring contraction.

Engage your hamstrings from a neutral pelvis position. This means avoiding an excessive anterior or posterior pelvic orientation while firing the hamstring. If the tendon is irritated, contracting the hamstring in a neutral position will decrease the pain.

90-90 Hip Lift

Lie on the ground and prop your feet up on a chair, coffee table, couch, or, if all else fails, the wall so your knees are at a 90-degree angle. Dig your heels into the ledge or surface your feet are resting on and feel your hamstring muscles engage. Using your hamstrings, tuck your hips under and scoop your pelvis up and off the ground (figure 13.7). Hold for five breaths, focusing on a strong exhale during which your ribs come down, in, and together. (This is important for maintaining a neutral pelvis.) Repeat three times, and aim to do this twice a day.

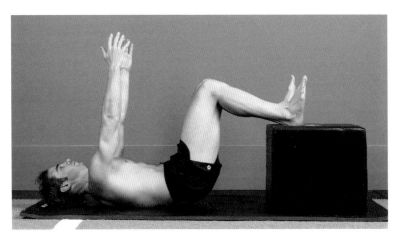

Figure 13.7   90-90 hip lift.

90-90 hip lift technique modified and used with permission. Copyright © Postural Restoration Institute® 2022. www.posturalrestoration.com.

Concentric Hamstring Strengthening

Once you've mastered isometric hamstring activation, the next step in rehab is concentric hamstring exercises (shortening of the muscle). Examples of concentric hamstring exercises include hamstring curls and dynamic bridges with double and single legs (versus the static isometric bridge holds described earlier). When appropriate, focus on co-contraction of the glutes and the hamstrings. The more the glutes and the hamstrings can function *together*, the more you can decrease the risk of injury to the hamstrings in running.

Hamstring Curl

Stand and lean against a wall or counter. Bend one knee, contracting the hamstrings to lift your foot up toward your butt (figure 13.8). In a slow, controlled motion, lower your foot back toward the ground. Repeat for three sets of 10. A theraband or ankle weights are a great addition and can be tolerated even early in the rehab program. For rehab purposes, you really only need to do this exercise on the injured leg, but you're welcome to do both legs if that makes the circuit feel more complete.

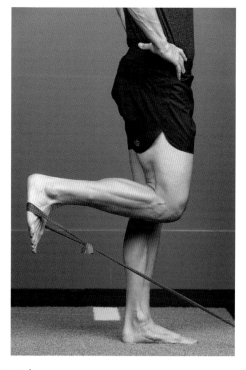

Figure 13.8 Hamstring curl.

Bridge

Lie on your back with knees bent. Tuck your hips underneath you so your back is pressed flat into the ground and abs are engaged. Press your heels and feet into the ground and push up into a bridge (figure 13.9). You should feel your hamstrings and glutes working. In a slow and controlled motion, lower back to the ground. Repeat 10 times.

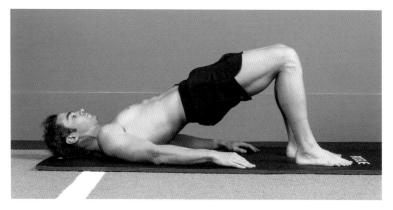

Figure 13.9   Bridge.

Once you can do this exercise easily with minimal or no discomfort (2 or less on the 1 to 10 pain scale), progress to single-leg bridges. Start by pushing up on two feet, lifting one leg off the ground, and then lowering down single-legged. If this is smooth and pain-free, then you can progress to doing the entire exercise with one leg (i.e., pushing up and lowering all on one leg).

Eccentric Hamstring Strengthening

Eccentric strengthening exercises are the third step. As discussed in chapter 1, eccentric muscle contractions involve the slow and controlled lengthening of a muscle under load, which helps to realign muscle and tendon fibers that have been damaged, as well as increase muscular hypertrophy (Bourne et al. 2017).

Double-Leg Towel Slide

Lie on your back, knees bent, with both heels on a towel. Push up into a bridge (figure 13.10a). Slowly slide the towel away as far as you can (figure 13.10b) and then back. You are controlling the extension of the hips and knees. Repeat 10 times. Once you can do this easily, with minimal or no discomfort (less than 3 on the 1 to 10 pain scale), progress to a single-leg towel slide.

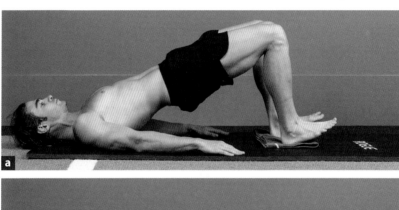

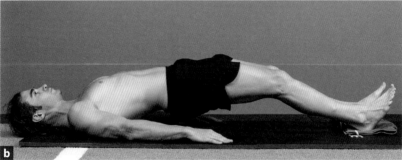

Figure 13.10   Double-leg towel slide: *(a)* push up into bridge; *(b)* slide towel away from body.

Single-Leg Towel Slide

Lie on your back, knees bent, with both heels on the towel. Push up into a bridge. Lift the unaffected leg to your chest (figure 13.11*a*). Slowly and with control, slide the heel of the leg you are rehabbing away from you (figure 13.11*b*) and then back. Repeat 10 times. Start with a small range (the leg does not need to go all the way to straight and back), and as you get stronger and your tolerance increases, you can progress to the full range.

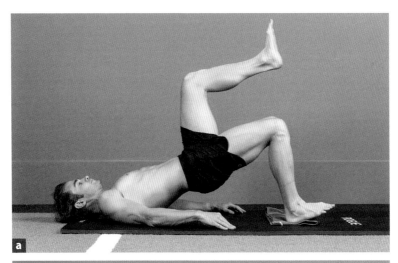

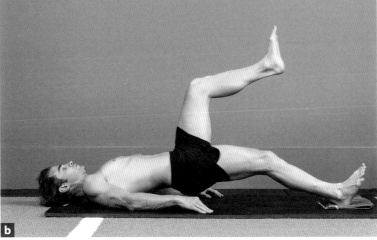

Figure 13.11   Single-leg towel slide: *(a)* lift leg in bridge position; *(b)* slide towel away from body with grounded leg.

Nordic Hamstring

Kneel on the ground with a partner behind you to hold your feet (figure 13.12*a*). Bending at the knees, try to lower yourself as far forward as you can control (figure 13.12*b*), and then come back to kneeling. Repeat 10 to 15 times.

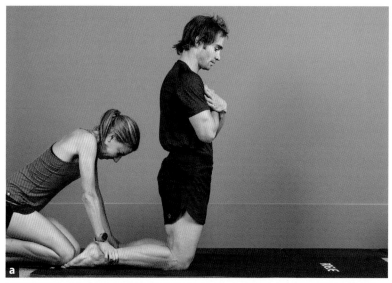

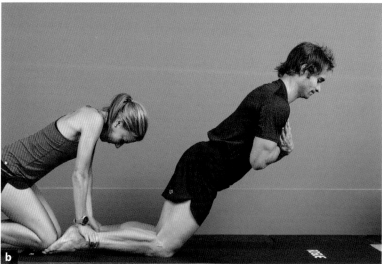

Figure 13.12   Nordic hamstring: *(a)* start position; *(b)* lower toward ground.

Hip Extension

This is an upgrade of the standard bridge. With your knees bent and your feet on an elevated surface (block, coffee table), push your hips up toward the ceiling (figure 13.13). Slowly come back down. Start with two legs, but once you can perform the exercise easily with minimum or no discomfort, progress to single leg. Once you've mastered single leg, progress to legs extended or straight (longer lever arm). Use a slow and controlled motion to come down.

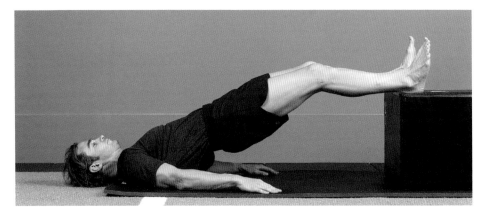

Figure 13.13   Hip extension.

Preventive Exercises

Even if you aren't rehabbing a hamstring injury, you can always do exercises to prevent one. We encourage you to choose from the following list of exercises. If you're trying them for the first time, check in with a movement professional to ensure proper form and mechanics.

In addition to the exercises described here, the Bulgarian single-leg split squat from chapter 7 and the common lunge matrix from chapter 8 are also great exercises for hamstring rehab.

Bridge With Feet on Foam Roller

Lying on your back, place both feet on a foam roller, knees bent to roughly 90 degrees (figure 13.14a). Push up into a bridge and hold (figure 13.14b). Start with 10 double-leg bridges, and then progress to performing the bridge with the foam roller farther and farther away from your butt until your legs are almost straight. Once you can do this without any pain, you can progress to single-leg bridges, again starting with the bridge at 90 degrees and progressively rolling the foam roller farther and farther away from your butt.

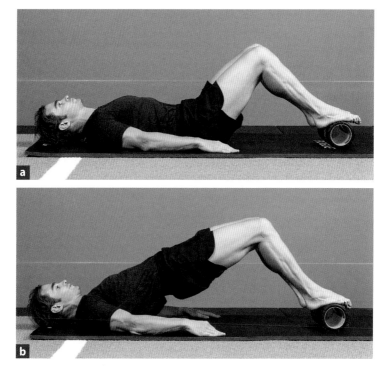

Figure 13.14   Bridge with feet on foam roller: *(a)* start position; *(b)* bridge.

Bridge Marches

This exercise is done lying on your back; you can do it with your feet on the ground, or on a foam roller for more difficulty. Push up into a bridge and alternate marching each leg off the ground (figure 13.15). Once you've mastered 20 reps, you can move your feet farther out to progress the exercise, similar to the Bridge With Feet on Foam Roller.

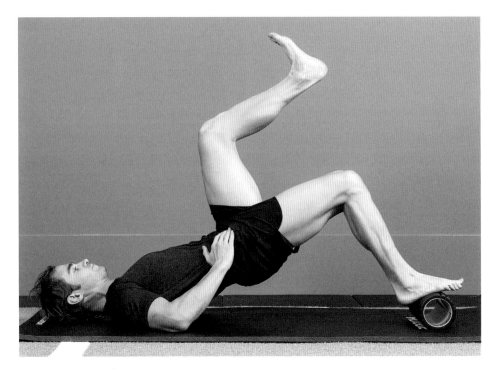

Figure 13.15 Bridge marches.

Hex Bar Deadlift

Although the classic deadlift uses a barbell, we prefer athletes use a hex bar because it lends itself to good form and prevents rounding the back. The exercise can also be done while holding a kettlebell in each hand.

Holding onto the bar or kettlebells, hinge your body forward (figure 13.16a). Pay attention to the hinge coming from the pelvis; you should feel this in the thighs, hamstrings, and glutes, *not* your back. Return upright (figure 13.16b). Once you can do 10 of these with proper form, you can increase the weight.

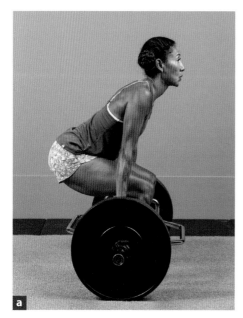 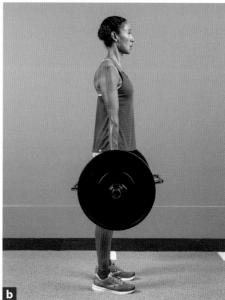

Figure 13.16   Hex bar deadlift: *(a)* hinge forward; *(b)* stand.

Single-Leg Romanian Deadlift

With dumbbells or a kettlebell in each hand and standing on one leg, hinge your body forward as with the traditional deadlift (figure 13.17). Your opposite leg will extend behind you. Make sure you keep your hips parallel so the opposite pelvis does not rotate away from your standing leg and extend up into the air. Once you can do 10 of these on each leg with very light weight, you can increase the weight.

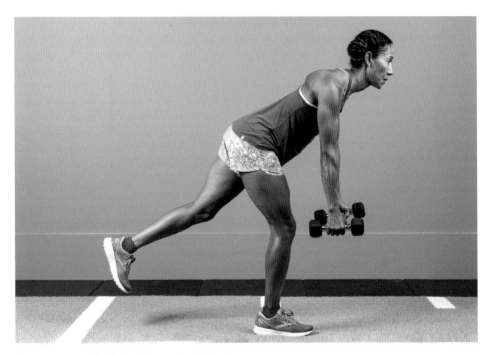

Figure 13.17   Single-leg Romanian deadlift.

Hip Thrust

Start seated on the floor with your knees bent, heels as close to your hips as possible, and your upper back against a bench (figure 13.18a). Ideally you will use a barbell with weighted plates on each side balanced across your hips, but you can also place a heavy kettlebell on your lap as a substitute. Thrust your pelvis up toward the ceiling so that your hips end in line with your shoulders and your knees, squeezing your glutes at the top (figure 13.18b). As your hips rise, your head and neck will tilt back until they're resting on the bench. You might feel a slight bounce in your hips as you push them upward; that's okay. Slowly lower your hips and repeat 10 times. When you can do this easily with good form, you can increase the weight.

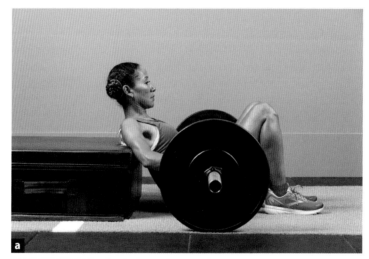

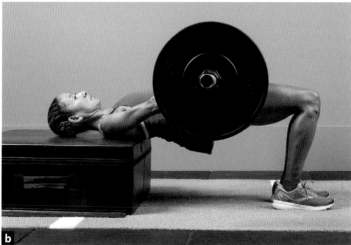

Figure 13.18   Hip thrust: *(a)* start position; *(b)* thrust.

Plyometric Training

The final stage in hamstring rehabilitation, or the icing on the cake of injury prevention, is plyometric training. Focused practice of A- and B-skips (see chapter 16), as well as jumping lunges, speed skaters, and double- and single-leg hopping drills, helps our bodies learn to engage our muscles dynamically—which has the added benefit of helping us run faster!

Form Specifics for Preventing Hamstring Injuries

Two things you can do to avoid putting excess stress on your hamstrings are controlling your running stride and activating and engaging your glutes prerun.

Overstriding is one of the most common running errors that leads to hamstring injury. This running position puts more force through the hamstring because you are requiring a very strong contraction from the muscle while in an overlengthened or stretched-out position. Two cues that can help with this are working on your cadence (shorter, quicker steps) and leaning forward from your ankles. Don't bend over; you want to think of shoulders, chest, hips, and legs being in a diagonal line as you lean. See chapter 16 for further description on proper running posture.

Performing glute activation exercises before your run, such as the lateral taps and monster walks in chapter 7 and the common lunge matrix and standing hip internal rotation in chapter 8, is a useful way to increase glute engagement while running. This preps your brain to use the hamstrings and glutes together to decrease the demands placed on your hamstrings, especially when moving at higher speeds.

Conclusion

If you take anything away from this chapter, know that hamstring injury prevention and rehab for runners is all about restoring neutral alignment of the pelvis and strengthening the hamstrings in this position. Avoid overstretching your hamstring, be mindful of cadence and posture, and activate those glutes before you head out the door, and you'll decrease your chances of hamstring injury.

CHAPTER 14

IT Band Syndrome

When a runner feels leg pain anywhere north of the calf or shin, one of the most common reactions is "I hope it's not my IT band!"

To understand how injury to the iliotibial band occurs, we first need to understand what this unique structure is, how it works, and the role it plays in running. The iliotibial band (IT band, or ITB) is a dense, long band of connective tissues, or fascia, located on the outer thigh and knee (figure 14.1). In fact, the ITB is the largest piece of fascia in the human body. Its role is similar to that of the Achilles tendon, functioning much like a spring or rubber band to help our hips and legs swing back and forth as we run. Evolutionary biologists believe the ITB to be an adaptation that came about from our two-footed locomotion, and it is essential for the conservation and efficient transfer of energy as we walk and run (Reuell 2015).

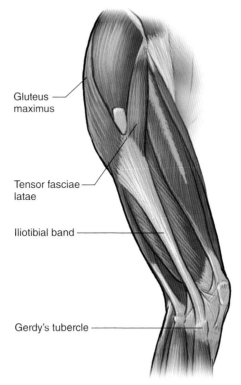

Gluteus maximus

Tensor fasciae latae

Iliotibial band

Gerdy's tubercle

Figure 14.1 Iliotibial band.

Causes of ITB Syndrome

So how does injury to the ITB, known as ITB syndrome, occur?

Despite years of research and several emergent theories, scientists have yet to reach a firm conclusion. The leading theories behind ITB syndrome are overuse, glute weakness, friction of the ITB gliding back and forth across the knee joint (lateral femoral epicondyle), or compression of the fat pad and bursae that lie underneath it (Fredericson and Wolf 2005; Hadeed and Tapscott 2020). Other factors leading to ITB pain can include overstriding, understriding, spending most of your day with your knee bent into flexion (sitting), or running on hills or uneven surfaces. Most likely, it's a combination of these factors that lead to ITB syndrome.

Hip mobility is a common root cause, so let's explore how this can lead to knee pain. Weak or tight hips affect how the femur moves inside the hip socket when the foot strikes the ground. In landing, the pelvis and femur move into flexion, adduction, and internal rotation as the head of the femur glides and spins backward in the socket. To learn more about hip movement and loading, refer to chapter 8.

This mechanism transfers the ground reaction force into the glute muscle, and the glute muscle uses this force to propel the runner forward. Think of it like a rubber band: On landing, the rubber band (glute) stretches and then recoils. Tightness in the hips and pelvis can limit this loading mechanism. Because the load (landing force) has to go somewhere, if it's not going into the glute, it's transferred into the side of the hip, namely the tensor fasciae latae (TFL) muscle.

A runner experiencing this problem might exhibit a lot of side-to-side motion (figure 14.2)—they are trying to use their TFL muscle the way the glute is designed to function. Unfortunately, the TFL is nowhere near as good as the glutes at accepting loads and generating power. If too much force and load are being put through the TFL, it will get overworked, tighten, and, in turn, restrict the movement of the ITB. A restricted ITB will cause friction and compression at the knee joint, resulting in "knee pain" that is ultimately diagnosed as ITB syndrome.

This can be a little bit confusing. You might ask, "All of this talk is about how the hip is loading, so why is it that my knee gets injured?" In short, the hip is the driver of the knee. Any tension or torque happening at the hip gets transferred down to the knee, so instead of feeling hip pain, the result is often lateral knee pain, because this is where the friction is the greatest. The hip joint is designed for rotation, whereas the knee joint is designed primarily to bend forward and backward; there isn't a lot of wiggle room for extra forces at this joint, so small rotational changes can cause irritation.

As a result, glute strengthening, hip mobilization, and running form improvements play a huge role in reducing lateral knee pain and preventing ITB pain from recurring.

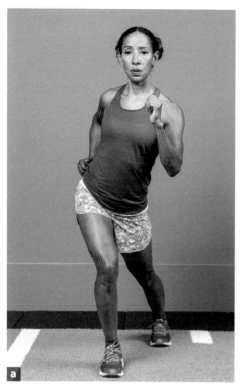 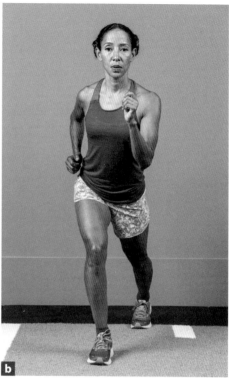

Figure 14.2 A runner who is experiencing *(a)* lateral versus *(b)* posterior loading into the hip joint.

Diagnosis

Now that we know what the ITB is and how it can be involved in injury, how can we determine if our knee pain is ITB syndrome or something else?

If the ITB is the culprit, you will feel pain on the *outside* of your knee and in movements where you bend your knee back and forth, like going up and down stairs or transitioning from sit to stand.

Other common sources of lateral knee pain that should be considered are a femoral stress fracture, lateral meniscus tear, knee arthritis, lateral collateral ligament strain, hamstring tendinitis, and patellofemoral syndrome. It can be difficult to distinguish between these injuries, so we recommend that you seek help from a medical professional if you are unsure or feel like the pain isn't getting any better after four to six weeks of modified activity and treatment.

Case Study: Soraya

Soraya was training for her first marathon when she began to experience acute knee pain. When she arrives at the physical therapist's office, she reports that she felt her knee locking up on her about three miles into her run, and once the pain started, it was difficult to continue running. On the days that she ran anyway, Soraya reports that she would have sharp pain every time she stood up from her desk and went down stairs; going up didn't feel great, but down was worse.

Observation: On assessment of Soraya's running form, we observe that she has excessive movement through her pelvis, with poor core and glute engagement when she runs. She presents with hip drop (figure 14.3), worse on the right side than the left. Her bad form is compounded by excessive internal rotation in her femur, again causing unstable and excessive lateral loading.

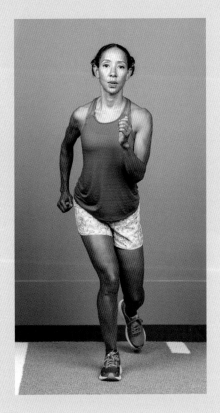

Figure 14.3 Hip drop.

Diagnosis: ITB syndrome driven by weak hips.

Treatment: After a few months of physical therapy, including myofascial decompression (cupping), core and glute strengthening, and running form corrections, Soraya is able to run the New York City Marathon pain-free.

Case Study: Michael

Michael was ramping up his running to cope with a stressful job; previously he had been an avid cyclist, but he was excited to try something different. Like Soraya, he comes in complaining of sharp pain on the outside of his knee. Michael also mentions that he had increased his weekday run distance from three or four miles to six to eight miles and had added a 12-mile run on weekends. He experiences pain both during his runs and throughout his workday. He also says that he has been struggling with the timing of his meals and maintaining a well-rounded diet.

Observation: When observing Michael's running form and movement patterns, we see that he demonstrates excessive external rotation of his femur, with increased internal rotation of his tibia and pronation of his foot as a compensatory movement. The exaggerated rotation is causing too much torque at his knee joint, and the resulting lateral pressure is contributing to inflammation of his ITB.

Diagnosis: ITB syndrome driven by hip tightness.

Treatment: Michael's physical therapist gives him daily movements to keep his knee from being in the flexed position for hours at a time at his desk, as well as a regimen of hip mobility exercises to work on his ability to rotate his pelvis correctly to diminish torque at the knee while landing, and strength to better control arch and foot pronation, as well as core and glutes. They also talk about his training routine—it's never a good idea to increase mileage abruptly, the way he had done. This holistic approach results in Michael healing his injury and remaining pain-free.

Soraya's and Michael's case studies demonstrate how two very different movement patterns can cause the same injury—and these are just two examples of many! While we hope the advice in this chapter can help you to relieve ITB pain, each and every body is unique; what has worked for friends, teammates, and even professionals may not work for you.

Treatment and Prevention

Now that we've covered the causes of ITB injury, let's talk about treatment and prevention. The first best strategy is always prevention. If you've struggled with ITB issues in the past, you know how debilitating they can be.

Foam Rolling

Keeping up with joint and muscle mobility both prevents and rehabilitates ITB injury. One treatment commonly recommended for ITB pain and injury is foam rolling. For those of you who have tried this, you know how much it hurts! But here's a secret: All that foam rolling is not doing anything to the ITB itself. It takes 2,000 pounds of pressure to make a 1 percent change to the length of the ITB; that's how strong this structure is (Chaudhry et al. 2008). The ITB is also highly innervated, which means two things: (1) foam rolling the ITB will hurt a lot, and (2) foam rolling the ITB is not going to improve the tension in the knee at all, unless your foam roller is a large cow walking on the side of your leg (and if that's the case, you might be holding a copy of the wrong book). Therefore, you'll gain the most from focusing on rolling and mobilizing the soft tissue structures that are attached to the ITB. Unlike the ITB itself, these structures do respond well to foam rolling because they contain muscle fibers, not connective tissue.

Because tightness in your TFL muscle can directly contribute to ITB syndrome, we recommend foam rolling the TFL, which is not made of the same ropey structure as the ITB itself. The TFL is the muscle that controls the tension in the fasciae, hence the name *tensor fasciae latae*. Translated from Latin, this literally means "stretcher of the side band." Unsurprisingly, stretching the "stretcher of the side band" muscle can help reduce the lateral stress on the ITB and its insertion. Your hamstring and lateral quad muscles also connect to the sides of the ITB, so these are good targets for foam rolling. Finally, some of the fibers of your glute muscle also attach to the ITB, so targeting these areas with the roller can be productive in alleviating tension at the knee (see foam rolling techniques for the glute, quads, and the TFL in chapter 8). Foam rolling these areas is often less painful than foam rolling the ITB itself.

Rest assured, if you have made a habit of religiously rolling out your ITB, you are not harming yourself, and some evidence points to the simple sensory input of the foam roller helping to reduce pain in the region. However, you may be more successful channeling your efforts toward the other areas we've just described.

Myofascial Decompression

You may have seen or heard of cupping, which is used in Eastern medicine practice and was made famous by Michael Phelps in the 2016 Olympics. While this treatment is touted for myriad benefits including pain management, blood flow, relaxation, and massage, it is used for a different purpose when treating ITB syndrome. Because ITB syndrome is a compression injury, the lifting and separating of the fasciae by decompression force (i.e., cupping) is an effective way to decrease the compression of the ITB as it glides across the knee joint. This decompression helps to relieve pain at the fulcrum of the injury and prevents excessive friction and compression at the joint by mobilizing the entire fascial chain and the muscles connecting to the ITB. It's somewhat intuitive; we want to decompress an overly compressed area. We can't lengthen or stretch the structure, but we can pull it apart.

It's not at all uncommon to see a physical therapist using a therapeutic plunger or cupping tools on the side of a leg or knee of a patient with ITB syndrome. However, before you go running to the bathroom to grab your plunger and "unclog" your knee, understand that this is a rather aggressive approach and not recommended to try at home. Instead, consult with a medical professional or licensed body worker to determine if this treatment could help with your specific injury.

Hip Mobility

The next key to ITB injury prevention and treatment is hip mobility. As we've described, tight hips limit the rotation, extension, and adduction of the pelvis and femur, meaning you won't be able to properly use your glutes when you run and will be prone to lateral loading. While glute strength is absolutely essential in the management and prevention of ITB syndrome, we first have to make sure that the pelvis can move in all three planes of motion so you can functionally access your glutes. Pelvic mobility exercises—common lunge matrix, 3D hip stretch, and 3D pivots—are described in chapter 8.

Hip Strengthening

Once we've gotten your hips moving correctly, we can start to talk about strengthening your glutes. Weakness and instability in the glutes can predispose a runner to overwork the TFL muscle, putting more tension through the side of the leg and the ITB. Remember, we want to increase the ability to load the hip with internal rotation (versus adduction) and help you keep the pelvis stable throughout the gait cycle. Therefore, while there are many exercises that strengthen the glute muscles, lateral toe taps (chapter 7) and the standing hip internal rotation lunge (chapter 8) focus on these specific functions of the glutes, which is why they are best for ITB rehab. We recommend including these two exercises as part of your pre-run warm-up if you are prone to ITB band syndrome.

Core Stability

Core stability also helps prevent and treat ITB syndrome. A lack of core stability can contribute to too much frontal plane (side-to-side) motion in the gait cycle or put the pelvis in a position that limits hip internal rotation. See chapter 9 for recommended core exercises for runners.

Training Considerations

Finally, all the strength and mobility in the world won't help stave off ITB syndrome if you don't integrate them into your form when you run. In fact, mobilizing your hips and strengthening your glutes is half the battle; making sure that you can engage your glutes more than your TFL when you run is equally critical. Practicing prerun hip mobility exercises and glute activation and focusing on leaning forward from your ankles while running can help with this. Again, no book can replace working with a running coach or movement professional on your form.

One final consideration is running cadence, or how quickly your feet hit the ground. An appropriately high cadence is important due to the sheer amount of friction going across the knee joint with each step. Having a higher cadence reduces the amount of impact that the knee is forced to absorb with each step. The ideal range is around 180 steps per minute.

Conclusion

We leave you with one final word of wisdom: If you are dealing with injury to your ITB, the most important thing you can do is *be patient*. This injury is slow to heal because of the nature of the ITB—it's built for strength, but without many blood vessels. To set yourself up for success, work on mobility and strength in the interim, while you are waiting for pain and inflammation to subside. Not only will this help to correct imbalances that caused your injury, but these exercises can help increase blood flow to the injured area, thereby expediting recovery.

PART IV

HEALTHY TRAINING

CHAPTER 15

Principles of Smart Training

The previous chapters of this book were dedicated to rehabilitating, treating, and minimizing the effects of running-related injuries—all of which is extremely important, given the high injury rate in our sport. However, the only thing better than bouncing back quickly from an injury is not getting injured in the first place. While we concede that some injuries are unavoidable, prudent training practices can help minimize the incidence of injury. One element of judicious training, in addition to strength and conditioning and mobility work, is a well-thought-out training plan.

The truth is that there are no absolutes when it comes to a running training program. What's optimal for one athlete will be too conservative for another and too aggressive for yet another. Still there are some common errors that we see far too often that lead to injury and that we can help you avoid. Runners who are trying to improve—and who isn't?—often fall into the trap of working too hard. That can mean overdoing it in a given workout, but more often it means pushing too hard on what should be an easy day, trying to build for too many consecutive weeks without adequate recovery, or trying to increase volume and intensity concurrently.

Ultimately, we always have to find a balance between risk and reward. An overly conservative training plan (e.g., with ample rest days, lots of low-intensity runs, and methodical increases in volume) is relatively safe but unlikely to have enough stimulus to elicit the improvements in cardiovascular fitness, running economy, and speed and endurance that you're seeking. Conversely, a program that features lots of hard days, little recovery, and an incessant pattern of increasing mileage will likely get results for a while but eventually lead to overtraining and injury, ultimately not getting you the results you're looking for, either. So while there's no-one-size-fits-all prescription for optimal training, there are certain principles that should be taken into consideration when designing a program that can maximize your chances of getting faster and remaining injury-free.

Periodization

The key principle of smart, effective training is periodization. Put simply, periodization is a systematic method of planning. Rather than haphazardly going out for a run with no purpose, a periodized training plan gives meaning and structure to each run, each week, each month, and each season. When properly developed and executed, periodization can help you peak at specific times of a season, while also incorporating extra recovery and rest at appropriate times of the year.

The reason periodization works is because it follows the body's stress–rest cycle. When training, we apply a stress to the body—in our case, in the form of running—and that stress produces an adaptation. When applied properly, the cycle is as follows:

1. Stress or training stimulus—during this time, you are adding new volume, intensity, or frequency to your training.

2. Fatigue as the result of the stress—during this time, performance level is diminished.

3. Recovery, often in the form of rest—during this time, tissues adapt to bear the stress in the future.

4. Supercompensation—during this time, performance level is higher than before the stress.

These four steps work as a cycle. This means that the process needs to continually start over for growth to occur. In other words, unless another stimulus is applied after the supercompensation, fitness will decrease.

In training, there are three variables that we can manipulate to elicit the desired stress: volume, intensity, and frequency. *Volume* refers to the amount of training. For runners, that means time spent running or distance run. Increasing your mileage is one simple way to increase the training stress.

Intensity refers to how hard the training stimulus is. Not all miles are created equally. An easy five-mile jog on flat ground is markedly different than a five-mile tempo run, five miles of hill work, or five miles of track intervals.

Finally, *frequency* is defined as how often the stimulus occurs. In running terms, this is often defined in terms of the number of days per week that you run versus rest or cross-train (more on cross-training later). For advanced runners or those pursuing high mileage goals, frequency can also include how many times you run in a day.

Together, volume, intensity, and frequency contribute to the totality of the training stimulus. If the stimulus is too low, it will not be great enough to cause significant improvement. Conversely, if it's too high, the fatigue will be too great, again stymieing improvement. The three variables are interdependent, so typically, if you significantly increase one, it makes sense to hold steady or decrease the others. Our experience training eager athletes, healing injured ones, and being athletes ourselves leads us to confidently say that while trying to increase all three elements at the same time may seem like the quickest way to get fit, it is a recipe for overtraining and injury and will not result in the performance gains you're seeking.

Annual Plan

To appropriately periodize your training, let's start with a bird's-eye view and look at a full season or, in periodization parlance, a macrocycle. Typically, within a given season, although you may race many times (depending on the distance of your race, as well as your necessary recovery time and other variables), it's only possible to truly be at your best, or "peak," two or three times within an annual macrocycle. Therefore, a common approach to structuring a macrocycle is to look ahead to a goal race—when you want to peak—and work your way back. For instance, if your goal race is the New York City Marathon in early November, you'll structure your training so that you peak on the first Sunday in November. Working backward, you have to decide: When would your taper begin? (Typically three weeks before race day.) When would the longest long runs need to happen? (Usually three and five weeks before the race.) When should you begin a specific marathon build from your base mileage? (In most cases, four months or so before race day.) At this point, you'll see that a good time to incorporate your base-building phase—consisting of more intense training where you work on physiological factors such as lactate threshold, $\dot{V}O_2$max, anaerobic capacity, neuromuscular integration, strength, and recovery—might be in the late spring and summer before your race, so that you'll be ready to start marathon training in July.

In sum, by first establishing a plan for a macrocycle, you can give meaning to each smaller phase of training.

Monthly Plan

Now let's zoom in a little from the macrocycle and look at a typical monthly plan, or *mesocycle*. Just as we have a structure and logic to the annual cycle, we lay out a month's cycle with an eye toward overall progress and include both hard and easy phases. A typical monthly plan will involve three weeks of building (intensity, mileage, or frequency), followed by one recovery week. The simplest form of a build could be an increase in volume: adding a few miles on week two, a few more on week three, and then backing off a little on week four. However, as with all these guidelines, this process is not written in stone. Some runners might hold steady on weekly volume for week four but cut out the midweek workouts (intensity) entirely. Another option would be to get away from the idea of a four-week cycle and do a three- or five-week cycle instead. Some athletes recover well and can handle a longer cycle (e.g., building for four weeks instead of three), while others tend to break down sooner and therefore benefit from a shorter cycle.

Many runners and coaches like to strictly adhere to the so-called 10 percent rule, which states that a runner should never increase their weekly mileage by more than 10 percent over the previous week's volume. While this is a nice guideline, there's a big difference between a relatively new runner making the modest jump from 15 to 16.5 miles and a grizzled veteran jumping from 90 to 99 for the first time. The former would not concern even the most conservative coach, while the latter is a definite red flag. While a 10-mile jump would be overkill for someone who hasn't been running for very long, bumping up weekly volume by 2 miles after a few weeks of training is perfectly reasonable. Thus, while the concept of not increasing too much too fast is a prudent one, there's no need to worry too much about exact percentages.

Weekly Plan

Now that we've looked at the training year and month, let's examine a typical training week, sometimes referred to as a microcycle in periodization-speak. In most cases, alternating easy and hard days works well. A standard training week might look something like this:

Monday: easy run, cross-train, or rest

Tuesday: track or other intervals

Wednesday: easy run

Thursday: tempo or hills

Friday: rest

Saturday: long run

Sunday: easy run or cross-train

Note how this plan splits up the challenging days, with at least one day of rest, cross-training, or easy running between them. That allows you to be relatively rested for—and therefore perform well on—those harder days. The most common error Coach Cane sees among underperforming runners is that their easy days are too hard. The result is often that the subsequent hard day is disappointing. In turn, the athlete feels guilty and frustrated, so once again pushes too hard on the next easy day and struggles again on the next hard day. Try to embrace the concept of easy days being easy so that hard days can be productive.

Of course, this weekly structure is not the only way. Some of Coach Cane's best athletes struggle with two "quality" sessions during the week when pushing the distance on their long runs. In cases like that, it's often best to do a single intense session on Tuesday or Wednesday, along with the Saturday long run, and complement those days with easy miles on the other days. Doing your long run on Saturdays, preceded by a rest day, is the most common protocol but not the only way to approach weekly scheduling. If you're training for a marathon and do all your long runs on relatively fresh and rested legs, conceptually you're preparing for the *first* miles of a marathon rather than the last. And since no one in the history of marathoning—from Pheidippides through Kipchoge—ever uttered the words "man, that first 10K was brutal, but things eased up after that" when referring to a marathon, some coaches (including Coach Cane) advocate for doing occasional long runs on fatigued legs by doing them on Sunday after a Saturday run or by running on the Friday before a Saturday long run in order to prepare for a marathon.

As you'd expect, the way you distribute these runs also depends largely on your goal event. A competitive miler will dedicate a greater percentage of training to higher intensity work, while a marathoner will emphasize a weekly long run and overall volume over speed. Unlike what you might expect, however, even a long-distance runner benefits from faster, quality miles, and even a miler can benefit from a relatively high volume of running. The weekly structure will usually be the same, though the distribution will vary.

Finally, the training stimulus doesn't necessarily need to be portioned out over exactly seven days. We call it a "weekly schedule," but for some athletes—and especially masters runners, who tend to need more time to recover—the "weekly" training cycle can be spread out over nine or more days. This gives the athlete more time to recover between bouts of acute stress (i.e., workouts).

Daily Plan

Now that we have an idea of how to lay out a season, a training month, and a training week, let's look at what makes up a single training session. Regardless of whether you're heading out for a long run, a tempo run, a track session, hill repeats, or an easy recovery run, there are certain aspects of the daily structure that should remain the same.

Begin with a warm-up. While certainly not the most glamorous part of a runner's routine, and one that many runners try to gloss over, it is vital from both an injury prevention and a performance perspective. Among other benefits, the warm-up literally raises your body temperature, delivering blood to the (soon to be) working muscles and lubricating your joints, therefore preparing you for a safe and effective workout. Dynamic movements such as leg swings (both back and forth and lateral), leg cradles, lunges, and 3D pivots are a good start. Then incorporate drills such as those outlined in chapter 16, and finally do some running, beginning at a low intensity and gradually increasing. Throwing in a few short strides is a good way to further increase your legs' range of motion and prepare for the run ahead. There's no need (and probably no value) to doing classic static stretches here. (More on that when we get to the cool-down.)

While it's tempting to skip the warm-up, it's also imprudent. On easy days, it's fine to do a few gentle dynamic movements and begin with an easy jog, but on more intense days, the warm-up needs to be more thorough. Forgoing the warm-up entirely decreases the effectiveness and the safety of the workout. (The classic analogy is a rubber band: A warm rubber band will stretch farther than a cold one, whereas the cold one is more liable to snap.)

After the warm-up is when you'll do the main part of the day's run—whatever that happens to be (intervals, tempo, active recovery, etc.). We'll come back to the specific types of workouts shortly.

When you finish the workout, it's time for the cool-down. As with the warm-up, the cool-down is often neglected by the time-crunched athlete, to that athlete's detriment. As the name suggests, the cool-down largely serves the opposite purpose of the warm-up. Remember how the warm-up brought blood to the working muscles? The cool-down helps redistribute your finite blood supply, since your muscles don't need it as much anymore, but your internal organs will benefit from getting some back. (When you finish running, blood and the metabolic byproduct of your intense effort, lactic acid, tends to pool in your legs unless you do an adequate cool-down to redistribute that blood. If you've ever felt lightheaded or dizzy when getting up from a seated position or lying down after a run, you've likely experienced orthostatic hypotension, which is a fancy way of saying that you had a drop in blood pressure brought on by a change in position and probably exacerbated by the blood pooled in your lower body.)

Typically, the more intense the run, the longer the cool-down. For instance, after an easy jog, just three to five minutes of brisk walking should be enough to do the trick, while a hard track session should be followed by at least one mile of easy jogging.

Sample Workouts

Let's dig a little into the nitty gritty of specific workouts. For a runner who races distances from the 5K to the marathon, a typical Tuesday track session might include a total volume of three to four miles at 5K to 10K race pace, broken into intervals and separated by recovery jogs. For instance, do five 1-kilometer runs at 5K race pace with 400-meter recovery jogs, or do four 800-meter runs at 10K pace with 400-meter recoveries, followed by four 400-meter runs at 5K pace with 200-meter recoveries.

Tempo runs are often referred to as "comfortably hard" or "brisk but sustainable." It's not race pace or even the pace you'd hit on a track, but it's not a leisurely jog, either. A typical tempo run might be four miles at half-marathon race pace, or three miles at marathon pace and two at half-marathon pace. (Of course, all workouts should be bookended by a warm-up and cool-down.)

Hill workouts are another example of quality runs and can sometimes be used in place of interval or tempo runs. A typical hill workout might be 4 to 8 repetitions up a 6 to 10 percent grade for two to three minutes with a slow jog down, to work on fitness; or 8 to 12 repetitions up a 10 to 15 percent grade for 30 seconds with a slow walk back down, to work on speed and biomechanics.

Last, we have long runs. For a miler or 5K runner, a long run of 10 to 12 miles every week or every other week is likely more than enough; alternatively, a marathoner would typically start their long run around 10 to 12 miles early in a marathon build and progress to 18 to 22 miles by the end of training. Generally, albeit counterintuitively, faster marathoners should usually do their long runs markedly slower than projected marathon race pace (30 to 45 seconds slower per mile), while those with more modest pace goals are better served sticking closer to marathon pace (up to 15 seconds slower per mile) in their long training runs.

The Value of Stretching

Many runners perform static stretching immediately after a run, and the ones who don't usually scold themselves for skipping it. But is there really a value in stretching?

Typically, the goal of just about anything a runner does is to improve performance, make them feel better, or decrease their risk of injury. To that end, since before anyone reading (or writing) this book was born, everyone from running coaches to high school physical education teachers to doctors and other health and fitness professionals has been recommending static stretching to runners.

Runners have been told to stretch to improve their speed, to decrease their risk of injury, to prevent soreness, to alleviate soreness, to improve economy, and just about any other reason imaginable. Classes have been taught and books have been written on the topic. Countless team practices have begun and ended with stretching sessions. Despite all that, the efficacy of static stretching, either as performance enhancer or injury preventer, is questionable, at best.

Let's take a closer look at why runners stretch, and whether they're really getting what they want and expect out of it.

Will Static Stretching Alleviate Soreness?

We've all woken up with some delayed onset muscle soreness (DOMS) a day or two after a hard effort. Almost instinctively, many of us begin stretching to ease or shorten the pain. Unfortunately, the truth is that a large body of research suggests that stretching does nothing to decrease the severity or duration of delayed onset muscle soreness (Herbert, de Noronha, and Kamper 2011).

Another common and persistent misconception is that lactic acid (or other mysterious and unnamed "toxins") need to be cleared from the body after exercise. On closer inspection, this one is at least a couple of steps removed from the truth. First, lactic acid isn't going to make your muscles sore after exercise (Schwane et al. 1983). Furthermore, lactic acid is removed from your body at the same rate, whether you stretch or not. If you're really anxious to get your lactic acid levels back down to baseline, an active cool-down (as advocated earlier) can help speed the process a little, but there's really nothing to worry about since one way or another, it'll be gone before too long (Menzies et al. 2010).

The good news (if there is any) is that as long as you stretch gently enough that you don't aggravate the already damaged tissue, stretching a sore muscle may feel good, in which case there's certainly no compelling argument against it. Just know what the stretching will, and won't, do.

Does Static Stretching Prevent Injury?

We've all heard that we should stretch because increased flexibility means decreased injury. But does it really? As you might imagine, stretching does increase flexibility. (Finally, some conventional wisdom that we're not debunking.) But will that make you a safer runner? According to Thacker et al. (2004), while stretching does improve flexibility, the highest quality studies show that the increased flexibility the stretching affords you probably won't do anything to decrease your chance of getting hurt. Actually, some research indicates that those who are overly flexible are as prone to injury as those with poor flexibility, while those with moderate flexibility are the least at risk. Jones and Knapik (1999) found that army soldiers with either high or low flexibility had injury rates more than double that of the "average flexibility" group. In other words, in the case of flexibility, more does not appear to be better with respect to injury prevention. Remember, a tight muscle, to a certain extent, is a strong muscle, and marathoners and ballerinas move very differently.

Of course athletes involved in sports that require extreme ranges of motion may have different results, so if you're a gymnast or a contortionist in the circus, by all means stretch, stretch, and then stretch some more. But for runners, it seems that stretching is not the injury prevention panacea we once thought.

Can Static Stretching Improve Performance?

Before just about every race you've ever done, you've probably seen runners touching their toes to stretch their hamstrings; standing on one leg, pulling up and back on the other foot to stretch their quadriceps; pushing against a tree to stretch the muscles of their calves, etc. That has to help them race faster, right? Sadly, no. In fact, probably quite the opposite. Numerous studies have shown that not only does stretching before a race not help performance, it may actually hinder it. For instance, one such study (Wilson et al. 2010) found decreased performance in stretching versus not stretching groups. Some research has even shown a negative effect on speed as a result of stretching for up to 24 hours after stretching (Haddad et al. 2014).

In addition, less flexible runners have been shown to have greater running economy than their more flexible counterparts (Craib et al. 1996). That means that at any given speed, the less flexible runner has a lower metabolic cost. While the physiological capacity of runners varies greatly, even the best physiological specimen will benefit from an improvement in economy, which suggests that increased flexibility is not necessarily advantageous.

Does this mean that stretching is of no value? Not necessarily. If a lack of flexibility leaves you with a limited range of motion in muscles needed to run effectively and efficiently, or you are unable to safely perform activities of daily living, by all means stretch. Just know what stretching can and can't do for you as a runner.

Flexibility Versus Mobility

Now that we've debunked the old way of thinking about static stretching, let's look at what might actually help you as a runner. Rather than focusing on flexibility, let's talk about mobility. Many times, you'll hear the two terms used interchangeably, but while they may be related, they are distinct and different attributes.

Flexibility is passive, while mobility is active. Flexibility uses external forces, such as body weight or gravity or a strap, to stretch. Think of grabbing the fingers of your left hand with your right hand and pulling the left hand as far back as it will go. You'll feel a stretch in the muscles of your wrist. That's demonstrating flexibility. Now, without the pull from your right hand, try to get your fingers as far back as you can using only the muscles of your wrist. Now you're demonstrating mobility.

Try this: Stand on one foot, engage the muscles of your core and hip flexors and raise your knee toward your chest. How high you can raise the knee is a measure of your hip mobility. Next, use your arms to hug your knee and pull it higher; that's demonstrating the flexibility of your hip. Mobility is active, flexibility is passive.

Similarly, you could have enough flexibility to do a split, but without the necessary strength to complement that flexibility, you won't be able to create adequate hip extension to create a long stride when running. Another way to look at this is our range of motion, and then our strength within that range. Having increased range of motion without control and strength within that range is an injury risk.

Flexibility is a prerequisite for mobility, but to have good mobility, you need to have strength as well. To promote mobility, focus on dynamic warm-up moves such as leg swings and lunges. If you want to do some gentle static stretches after the dynamic warm-up, that's fine, but you can feel guilt-free if you forgo them.

An ideal warm-up routine starts with foam rolling any areas that feel a bit tight or problematic. Next, follow with a dynamic warm-up. The 3D pivots and the common lunge matrix described in chapter 8 are great for global, triplanar mobilization. Following the dynamic warm-up, spend a few minutes activating muscle groups that play an important role in injury prevention using lateral toe taps (chapter 7) and the runner's lunge (chapter 9). Now you're on your way! Begin with an easy jog, then top it off with drills and strides, and you are ready to crush your workout. This ideal warm-up is not critical for easy runs every single time you step out the door, but stick to it on your quality and intensive days.

For cooling down, continue moving for a time to facilitate blood flow to the muscles that were just working hard, which can help to flush out the body posttraining. Pace absolutely *does not matter*. For some runners, cool-down effort may even be a walk, and that is okay; we just recommend that you continue to move for 15 to 20 minutes after a hard effort. Follow with foam rolling on any areas that feel tight and any of your favorite, gentle stretches. Finally, don't forget about proper hydration and postexercise fueling (depending on the length and intensity of the effort).

Cross-Training

Depending on the type of athlete you are, you either look forward to or dread your cross-training days. While a lot of runners look at cross-training as time away from the sport they love (and many have experienced cross-training as simply a means of maintaining fitness while injured), cross-training can be a valuable tool for runners. Non- or low-impact activities such as cycling and swimming, for instance, can provide a stimulus for cardiovascular benefit without the orthopedic stress associated with running. As such, these activities work well for a runner returning from injury or whose body is showing signs of needing a little break. Of course, if your goal is to run a fast mile, 5K, 10K, half-marathon, or marathon, running should be the main weapon in your training arsenal, but it need not be the only one. Coach Cane, who coaches many triathletes, as well as runners, has often transitioned athletes from triathlon to running training by having them run quality workouts and long runs, but complementing those with some swimming and cycling for a while as the athlete gets acclimated to higher mileage. This strategy can also work well for runners who are coming back from injury or a break or who are training for longer races but are injury-prone.

Strength Training

Given that it's not running, strength training is a form of cross-training; however, unlike swimming, cycling or other forms of optional aerobic exercise, strength training is essential to being a well-rounded, injury-resistant athlete.

You may hear about strength work in the context of trying to make healthy runners faster. The focus is often on strengthening the prime movers, such as the hamstrings, quadriceps, and glutes, to improve performance. In fact, the jury (if the jury were made up exclusively of exercise scientists) is still out on whether stronger muscles translate directly to faster running. It appears that if improvements in performance are seen, they're due to improved running economy, rather than changes in physiological variables such as $\dot{V}O_2$max or lactate threshold (Jung 2003). Strength training does not make you a faster runner, but strength training makes you more resilient, so your body can better handle the demands of training with decreased chance of injury. You're increasing your buffer zone.

The authors, an exercise physiologist and a physical therapist, feel strongly that strength work is important for runners. Addressing muscular weaknesses and imbalances can help prevent or minimize injuries, further improving overall performance due to fewer missed training opportunities.

Frequency

Before we dive into the specifics of what, when, how, and why, allow us to answer a common question asked by runners who would rather be running than doing virtually anything else: "How often do I have to strength train?" The short answer is that while it depends on your goals, you do not need to strength train as often as you might think. Coach Cane often refers to the off-season as the time to get strong, while the goal for his athletes in-season is to maintain those off-season strength gains. Typically, that can be accomplished by two or three sessions per week during the off-season and one session every 7 to 10 days in-season. While it may seem preferable to strength train more often, recognize that muscles need time to recover from the stress of training. For racers, the in-season schedule probably needs to be adjusted periodically to prioritize running and racing, but surprisingly little volume is needed to hold on to the strength gains developed during higher-volume phases. These guidelines are for a healthy runner; if you are rehabilitating from an injury, specifically a tendon injury, even during the on-season, two or three times a week may be necessary.

Form

Now that we have frequency out of the way, let's move on to the absolute most important aspect of strength training for runners. Given that this book's primary purpose is to help you treat and prevent injuries, safety is paramount at all times when doing strength work. After all, getting hurt performing an exercise that's supposed to keep you healthy defeats the purpose. And the number one thing you can do to ensure your safety when strength training? *Maintain proper form.*

If you are an uber-competitive runner, prioritizing form often means checking your ego at the door. Compete on the racecourse, not in the weight room. We'd much rather you use 50 pounds for an exercise and perform it with pristine form than use 75 or 100 pounds for the same exercise but compromise your form. Not only does compromising form increase your chances of getting injured, it also decreases the effectiveness of the exercise.

What do we mean by *form*? What we don't mean is to mimic a competitive powerlifter. While we can learn from athletes in other sports, emulating an Olympic weightlifter is not prudent. Moving weight from point A to point B is the stated goal of their sport, and therefore their job is to do anything within the rules to accomplish that. Such techniques include holding their breath (technically referred to as the *Valsalva maneuver*, which can be very dangerous because of the effects on blood pressure), using momentum to help move the weight past sticking points where they're not as strong, and other tried-and-true tricks like using incomplete range of motion. That competitive lifter is doing everything within their power to make it as easy as possible to execute an exercise, but your goal is the opposite. Their goal is to *demonstrate* strength, while your goal is to *gain* strength. So never try to squeeze out an extra repetition or add a few pounds of resistance if it comes at the expense of form or safety.

Often we see athletes who are preoccupied with numbers rather than form. If you can't properly execute more than a few perfect push-ups, don't opt for incomplete range of motion or extended breaks at the top with your elbows locked just for the sake of doing a set of 10. Instead, be smart and modify the push-ups by bending to your knees. That effectively decreases your resistance and will make it easier to get your chest down to the floor. More importantly, it will allow you to start gaining strength through that full range of motion (ROM); that is, the full extent of an exercise, from beginning to end. Because muscles only get strong through the range of motion in which they're trained, doing shallow push-ups with limited ROM will get you better at doing push-ups with limited ROM, but it won't have much of an effect through the range of motion you've neglected.

Weight Room Terminology

To feel comfortable in the weight room, learn some of the terminology used to describe strength training exercises and sessions.

Range of Motion (ROM)

As we have said, range of motion is key to good form and often gets sacrificed as an exercise becomes harder. In most cases it's best to work your muscles through their full ROM in order to maximize strength gains. For instance, a wall sit is a perfectly useful exercise for treating patellar tendinitis and PFPS, but for general strength gains, use lunges, squats, or other movements that work your muscles through a wider ROM.

Repetitions

Executing one exercise one time is referred to as one repetition, or rep. It is essentially the smallest unit of an exercise. A competitive lifter's goal is to maximize their one-repetition max (1RM), or the amount they can lift one time. For runners, that's not of any concern and not something we need to test. Focus on doing all you can to ensure that the form for every single repetition you do is safe, correct, and as close to identical as possible.

Sets

A group of repetitions performed continuously is known as a set. For instance, you might do a set of 10 reps before stopping. If you do that and then repeat it, it's two sets of 10 reps, or what would typically be notated as "2 × 10." Generally speaking, we want most of your sets to be in the 8- to 12-repetition range unless otherwise noted.

Volume

The number of sets you do in a workout is referred to as the volume. We typically advocate a relatively low volume for runners to ensure you don't take too much time away from your running. In other words, rather than doing four or five sets per exercise, we usually prefer one or two sets. There are a few justifications for this strategy. First, the muscular strength and endurance gains from either low- or high-volume scenarios are comparable. Of note to runners, who often express concerns about bulking up from strength training, there is evidence that the additional sets (which, as noted, do not contribute to additional strength gains) do lead to greater increases in muscle size (hypertrophy; Schoenfeld et al. 2019). Plus, there's the obvious advantage that less volume takes less time.

Resistance

Resistance can take numerous forms. Most simply, it's weight (such as a dumbbell, barbell, kettlebell, or even your body weight) that you move against the force of gravity. But it can also be a band or weight plates or pneumatic resistance on a machine. There are advantages and disadvantages to each, but for the most part, if it makes your muscles work hard, it has value.

Generally, start by erring on the side of minimal resistance when you're learning a new exercise or returning to one you haven't done in a long while. The reason is to begin by practicing perfect form, of course. Once you're able to perfectly execute the maximum number of prescribed repetitions, it's time to make a small increase in resistance, about 5 percent or so. Conversely, if you can't do the minimum number without sacrificing form, it's best to decrease the resistance.

Intensity

Intensity is a tricky variable to measure, but it is key nonetheless. Unlike amount of resistance or number of repetitions, which are easily quantifiable, judging intensity is hard. In theory, all you can accurately identify is zero, in which you're doing nothing, or 100 percent, in which you're working as hard as you can.

If you don't pass a certain threshold of intensity, you won't recruit a significant amount of muscle fibers and gain strength. Therefore, we want you working hard—close to 100 percent by the final repetition of a set—but not so hard that you sacrifice form or safety.

Speed of Movement

A common misconception is that faster movements preferentially recruit fast-twitch muscle fibers and increase speed. In fact, muscle fibers are always recruited in an orderly fashion, from slow-twitch to fast-twitch, regardless of the speed of movement. To that end, therefore, faster is not better. Additionally, how fast you overcome a given resistance can impact how challenging it is. Faster movements generally allow for the use of momentum and can make an exercise easier. Speed can also make the exercise less safe. Consequently, we advise focusing on performing most movements slowly and under control.

Exercise Selection

The choice of what exercises to do affects the efficacy of your strength program. Select exercises that strengthen the muscles that help propel you but also work on core strength and the stabilizing muscles that will help limit extraneous movements. Throughout the book, you'll have seen some exercises that favor certain motor patterns and use all three planes of motion and some exercises that emphasize strength gains.

If you're doing exercises for therapeutic reasons, you'll obviously prioritize them. If you're training for general fitness, you're likely best served by performing exercises that address multiple joints and big muscles first (such as squats and deadlifts) and then progressing to ones that work smaller muscles (such as shoulder presses). Here are some of the exercises we recommend most often to our healthy athletes looking to gain strength and prevent injury:

- Bulgarian single-leg split squat (chapter 7)
- Deadlift (chapter 13)
- Hip thrust (chapter 13)
- 3D plank with hip drivers (chapter 9)
- Side plank elbow to knee (chapter 10)
- Push-up or pull-up (with modifications if necessary for proper form)

Conclusion

As always, there is no one-size-fits-all recommendation that is perfect for every runner, but the guidelines presented in this chapter should help you formulate a game plan to maximize your potential, as well as avoid unnecessary and ineffective methods. We encourage you to customize your training program to suit your needs but try to embrace these foundational concepts to build a smart training program that keeps you healthy.

CHAPTER 16

Ideal Running Form

The title of this chapter, Ideal Running Form, is slightly misleading. Really, there's no such thing as ideal running form. In fact, some of the greatest runners could have been featured in a textbook on how *not* to run. Take Pat Petersen, the former Manhattan College great, with three top-five NYC Marathon finishes on his résumé. After his death, *Runner's World* magazine wrote, "His running style also attracted attention, much of it negative. It was an ungainly, arms-flailing motion that one reporter described as 'awful'" (Hanc 2015). Yet, as the story goes, every time a coach tried to "fix" Petersen's stride, his times deteriorated.

Another chapter in the "bad form, fast runner" book could be dedicated to former world record holder Paula Radcliffe, who looked like she had a chronic case of hiccups when she ran. Her form might not have been enviable, but it worked for her—she won the New York City and London marathons three times each. So while maybe we can't learn from her form, we can learn that the notion of ideal form is flawed.

Indeed, one of the great things about running is its purity. Running is not gymnastics or diving or figure skating. There are no style points awarded, no bonuses for artistic interpretation. The first runner across the line wins. Period.

Good Form Practices

Nevertheless, there are certain concepts and practices that we like runners to keep in mind. Doing so can help contribute to making you a more mechanically sound and efficient runner, and it may help keep you off the sidelines, as well.

The short version is fourfold:

1. Stay relaxed but firm.
2. Don't waste energy on extraneous movements.
3. Maintain a subtle forward lean.
4. Have your feet land gently beneath your center of gravity.

These concepts all sound fairly simple, but putting them into practice can be tricky. Plus, we want you to understand why they're important and how they'll help you. Therefore, let's go into a little more detail, working our way from head to foot.

Head and Neck

Start by maintaining a long spine (figure 16.1). You can do this by picturing a helium balloon gently pulling up through the center of your head. Another common cue is to "run tall." This cue helpfully instructs you to lengthen your spine and maintain good posture; however, it's slightly misleading, because rather than staying ramrod straight up and down, you want to maintain a slight forward lean. This does not mean to hunch over; lean from the ankles rather than the waist. In other words, take that tall body and hinge forward at the ankles by a few degrees. Doing this helps to engage your glutes and enables your core muscles to work to your best advantage.

Other than that, keep your head up and chin gently tucked (rather than protruding forward). A lot of runners fall prey to the posture-killing habit of looking at their feet when they run. Unless you're on technical trails, there's no value in doing this. As Coach Cane's longtime coworker Shane Neil used to say, "There are no landmines on the track." Look where you're going—not where you are.

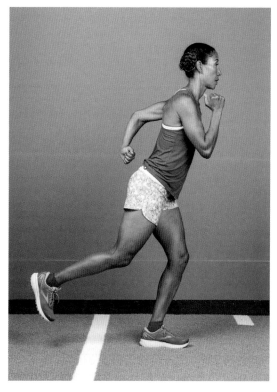

Figure 16.1   An example of running tall.

Shoulders

Your shoulders should be relaxed and square or facing forward, not hunched over. Not only are hunched shoulders generally bad posture for life, but rounding the shoulders too far forward tends to tighten the chest and restrict breathing. You'll breathe a lot easier if your shoulders are relaxed, and goodness knows, the easier you can breathe on a run, the better that run will feel.

The other shoulder mistake runners often make is to start pulling their shoulders up, or shrugging, when they start getting tired. Doing so may feel benign at first but can eventually cause pain in your shoulders and neck. Plus, your shoulders are not connected to your feet, so lifting them higher won't keep your feet moving! Start paying attention to how your shoulders feel on your runs, and if you notice they've snuck up, intentionally lower them and gently squeeze your scapulae (shoulder blades) together—down and back.

Arms

When you're running, your legs do a lot of the work, but your upper body also helps propel you. Typically, the shorter the distance, the more you'll use your upper body; sprinters swing their hands from down at their waist up to their faces, while marathoners typically have a much smaller movement, in order to conserve energy. Still, both need that arm swing to move.

Regardless of the degree to which you're using your upper body, make sure that you are pivoting from your shoulder joint rather than your elbow (figure 16.2*a* and figure 16.2*b*). Movement (extension and flexion) at your elbow joint will generally result in wasted energy. Therefore, aim to keep your elbows bent to about 90 degrees, and maintain that position rather than "karate chopping." Your upper arm should stay close to your torso, possibly even brushing against it. Helpful cues to facilitate proper shoulder movement are "reach forward" and "drive your elbow backward."

Finally, avoid too much side-to-side arm swinging. If your hand crosses your midline, it will likely take the opposing leg with it to counteract that lateral movement, resulting in wasted movement and energy (because remember, you're trying to move forward, not side to side). One way to help prevent this is to stick out (or imagine sticking out) "hitchhiker's thumbs" from each hand. This rotates your forearm slightly outward so your wrist is facing the sky and makes it much harder to swing your arms across your body.

Hands

Keep your hands relaxed as you run. Don't clench your fists, because the tension is wasted energy and typically works its way up your arms to your shoulders and neck. A common cue to prevent tight fists is to imagine that you are holding potato chips between your thumbs and index fingers, and you want to finish your run with the chips intact.

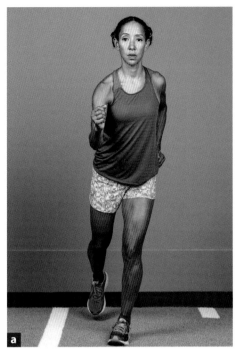 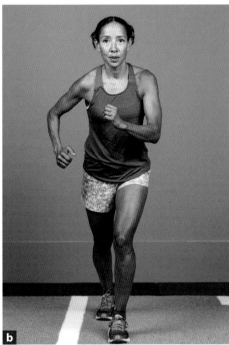

Figure 16.2   Arm motion: *(a)* runner with good form (elbows bent, arms tight to the sides, no lateral crossover); *(b)* runner with poor form (swinging from the elbow instead of the shoulder, arms crossing the midline).

Abdomen or Core

This is an area that often gets ignored when discussing form, perhaps because of the Goldilocks complex that goes along with it. You need to find a happy balance between too relaxed and too tense with your abdominal muscles. If they're too relaxed, your body will become unstable and you'll flail around (think of the blow-up character at the local car dealer), making extraneous movements that waste energy. On the other hand, this is running, not boxing, so unless you expect a right hook from the runner next to you, there's no need to have your abs fully contracted at all times. Aim to stay firm and stable, but not overly tense—again to avoid unnecessarily wasting energy.

The other thing to mention is the difference between your rectus abdominis (i.e., six-pack muscles) and your obliques. In running, the rectus abdominis is, comparatively, just for show; these muscles are up and down the front of your body, and they don't do much to help you move forward. On the other hand, the obliques, the muscles that wrap around your waist, are the real workhorses. While you naturally run with "opposite arm, opposite leg," your obliques work in opposition to your glutes to rotate your body and slingshot you forward. All of which is to say: Strong obliques are key to good form!

Hips and Pelvis

Discerning the placement of one's own hips can be challenging, but if you're generally "tight" in and around your hips, and especially if you're experiencing chronic injuries, it's worth seeing a professional to suss this out. In a nutshell, your pelvis needs to have adequate rotation to help with the load and explode phases of the running cycle. When you land, the pelvis rotates backward as the femur loads into the hip socket, stretching or "activating" the glute. Then, as you push off, the glute works like a rubber band, propelling you forward as the hips rotate forward.

Proper hip mobility is critical for runners, and an area that is often lacking—which is a big contributor to injury. A common issue among many runners is having hips that are stuck in forward rotation, or anterior pelvic tilt (see figure 16.3). While some anterior tilt is necessary, having really tight hip flexors can pull the pelvis too far forward, which, from an injury risk point of view, can create excess strain on the hamstring muscles (which attach to the back of the pelvis), inhibit the glutes from functioning properly, and cause excess stress on the low back. And even if you've escaped injury, excessive anterior pelvic tilt will affect your performance, as well, by limiting your ability to create knee lift in your stride.

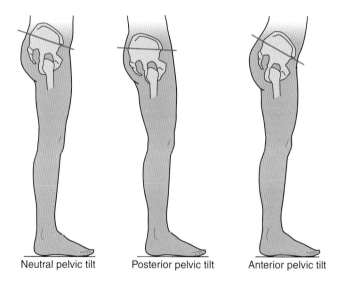

Neutral pelvic tilt   Posterior pelvic tilt   Anterior pelvic tilt

Figure 16.3   Runner displaying neutral, posterior, and anterior pelvic tilt.

Feet

While many coaches like to tell runners what part of their foot (heel, midfoot, forefoot) should strike the ground first, we see that as "the tail wagging the dog." Instead, we guide runners to focus on other factors in their running form and then let the foot strike work itself out. So, what are those other factors? There are several, but the primary one that affects the others is foot placement, or where your foot is landing relative to your center of gravity.

To get a feel for how foot placement affects foot strike, try running in place. You'll notice that you're landing gently on your forefoot or midfoot, and landing on your heel is almost impossible. Conversely, if you are walking and take the longest stride possible, you'll no doubt land hard on your heel and will be unable to get your toes down first.

We'll soon share running drills to help encourage a cycling-like stride that will get your foot to land gently under your center of gravity. For now, let's consider why this type of stride makes sense, as well as what it has to do with your foot strike. Specifically, we'll examine how your stride should *not* look—that is, what it looks like when you overstride.

Overstriding essentially means landing with your foot too far in front of your center of gravity (see figure 16.4*a* and figure 16.4*b*). It's counterproductive in that it slows you down because your foot spends too much time on the ground. Also, it leads to landing with an extreme heel strike and straight(er) knee, which in turn creates a lot of impact that can lead to injuries.

To avoid overstriding, there are two variables to consider. The first is your stride rate. Many runners use a lower-than-optimal stride rate and, as a result, have an overly long stride. For years, runners heard coaches say that 180 strides per minute is ideal, but that's actually a big oversimplification. A runner's pace and size, among other considerations, affect their ideal cadence. However, if you notice that you're overstriding, a good first step (pun intended) is to subtly increase your stride rate by two or three strides

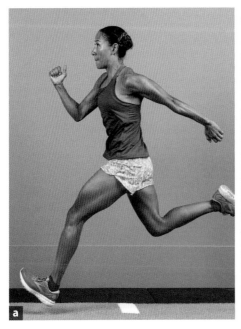 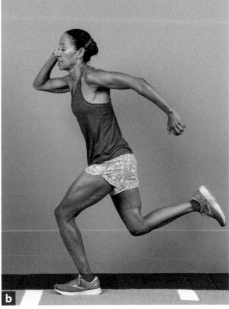

Figure 16.4 *(a)* Overstriding with heel strike versus *(b)* landing under center of gravity on the midfoot.

per minute. Unless you have energy to spare, you'll need to decrease your stride length in order to keep your speed constant as you do this, which can keep you from reaching too far out in front of you with each footfall.

The other variable to consider is the actual mechanics of your stride. Tell a runner to increase their stride length, and the first thing they'll do is land with their foot way out in front of their center of gravity, but what we really want to see is greater hip extension. In other words, as your stride gets longer, we still want to see your foot land gently beneath your center of gravity, so instead of lengthening by reaching out in front, your foot will extend farther *back* with each stride.

Increasing your hip extension and cadence, as appropriate, contributes to eliminating overstriding, which, in turn, leads to your foot landing under your center of gravity. What you'll notice when you follow this advice is that you no longer have that counterproductive, pronounced heel strike that you always hear about. Ergo, you focused on your form, and your foot strike worked itself out—just like we promised.

Many playlists available online feature songs with set cadences. Using these playlists can help you increase cadence, and your running watch can help as well. If you're averaging 150 steps per minute on most runs, it doesn't make sense to try to jump straight to 180. Rather, find a playlist that targets 155 to 160 beats per minute (one beat per footfall), and work your way up gradually. To avoid overstriding when increasing stride length, think about picking up your knees or driving your knees forward. In addition to running drills, this can be a great cue to even out your gait cycle and keep your foot landing underneath you.

Drills to Improve Form

As we have already discussed, there's no one perfect form for every runner. Still, you can practice certain techniques and drills to make you run faster and more economically and, quite possibly, make you less prone to injuries. Drills typically emphasize or exaggerate a particular aspect of the running stride to help you notice, feel, and improve it. They can also help to develop the neuromuscular aspects of running—that is, the connection between your brain and your muscles—so that elements of your stride you initially have to focus on eventually become natural and automatic.

Drills also help you become a more efficient runner. From an exercise physiology point of view, you'll have greater running economy—in other words, you can run faster without getting any fitter. That means faster sprinting at the end of a race, or a faster sustained speed during a race, without any change in your $\dot{V}O_2$max, lactate threshold, or other physiological parameters.

Now that we've made our compelling case and convinced you that you should do drills, let's discuss which ones. Just as a doctor wouldn't walk into the waiting room, look at all the patients, and say, "Here's my favorite prescription, you should all take it," not every drill is right for every runner. However, a doctor *would* tell everyone in the waiting room to get seven to nine hours of sleep and to eat more vegetables; similarly, there are some universal drills that are appropriate regardless of your current form or speed. Adding these to your routine can help make you faster, more efficient, and healthier.

High Knees

The high knees drill is perhaps the most common running drill—and for good reason. It helps your front-end mechanics, discourages an overly harsh heel landing, works on hamstring mobility, and (especially when paired with the butt kick drill that appears next) encourages a high cadence, with your foot landing gently beneath your center of gravity.

Stand tall but do not lean back. Lift the knee of your lead leg until you have a nearly 90-degree angle at your knee (figure 16.5). Lower your leg, focusing on a light forefoot landing with your foot dorsiflexed, and switch legs. (Dorsiflexion simply means bending your ankle back. Think of the last time you were speeding and saw a police car ahead. When you pulled your foot off the gas, you dorsiflexed your ankle.) As with running, coordinate your opposite arm with your leg. The hand should come up to your chin when the knee is up, and down to your hip when the leg is straight.

When doing a high knees drill, the goal is to get your upper leg parallel to the ground. While a distance runner would rarely, if ever, have the need to raise their knee this high, practicing this exaggerated knee lift is particularly useful if you've ever found yourself dragging your feet or if you have an overly short stride.

There are a few variations on the high knees drill, but each of them focuses on (as the name suggests) getting your knees up. Rather than simply jumping right into the full drill, we recommend progressing through a few variations until you become comfortable with the movement. Aim to do each variation for 10 to 15 seconds (which we'll count as a set), and perform two or three sets. Allow ample recovery between sets, and if you find your form deteriorating, reset, rest, and start again. Because of the neuromuscular aspect of this and other drills, it's counterproductive to do them with bad form.

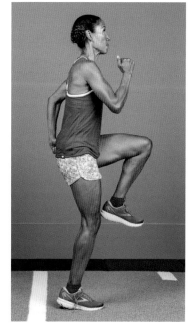

Figure 16.5   High knees.

Marching

Start your high knees drill progression by marching at a deliberate pace that allows you to focus on your body position and the movement (figure 16.6). Be slow and deliberate, paying close attention to position and alignment. (The most common form error we see is runners leaning back rather than standing tall.)

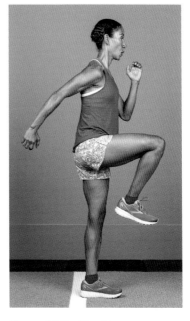

Figure 16.6   Marching.

A-Skips and B-Skips

A-skips (figure 16.7) are essentially a variation of the marching stage of the high knees drill. The start and finish positions are the same (one leg at 90 degrees, the other straight), but the cadence is faster, and you do a quick skip off the stance leg as you lift the opposite knee (as opposed to marching, where that stance leg stays rooted to the ground). What you're focusing on is the rebound of your foot as it strikes the ground and quickly comes off again—the impact should involve the posterior chain of muscles (glutes, hamstring, and calf). Begin by doing the skips in place, and progress to moving forward.

B-skips are variations of A-skips where,

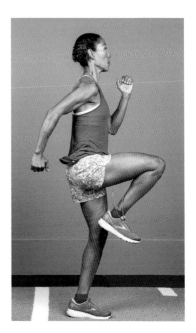

Figure 16.7   A-skip.

instead of bringing your raised foot down directly beneath you (as you would in a march), you *extend* the leg on its way down (figure 16.8*a* and figure 16.8*b*). Think of clearing a hurdle with that lead leg and then quickly "snapping" the leg down. You are not dancing the can-can, so don't kick that leg out; you're trying to activate your hamstrings and glutes, so you want the movement to imitate scraping gum off the bottom of your shoe. (If you picture a horse pawing the ground, that'll also give you the right idea for the motion. Horses don't dance the can-can!) Another cue is where your foot is landing: If it's in front of you when it hits the ground, you're doing the drill incorrectly. Your foot should land beneath your body, just like when you're running.

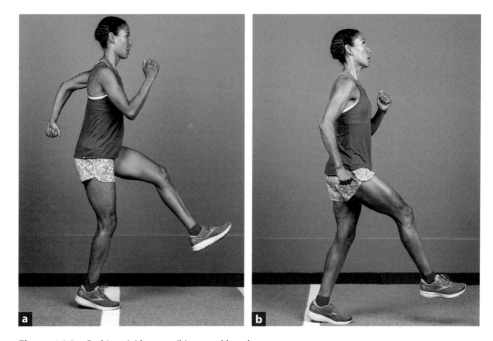

Figure 16.8   B-skips: *(a)* leg up; *(b)* extend leg down.

Running

Once you've reached a level of confidence and comfort with the marching and skipping, the final step is the full high knees drill with no skipping and no pausing. Simply perform a quick alternating stride emphasizing a powerful lift, followed by an active, driving downward motion.

Butt Kicks

Butt kicks are a nice complement to high knees. Together they promote a cycling-like motion of your legs, with your foot strike occurring under your center of gravity and your foot moving backward. Butt kicks are great for improving hip extension by encouraging quadriceps and hip flexor flexibility. This means that if you increase your stride length, it can be done through greater hip extension rather than by having your foot land well forward of your center of gravity. Your speed is a function of stride rate and stride length. If rate stays the same and length increases, your speed will increase too. An increase in stride length needs to come from greater extension (i.e., the back of the stride) rather than having your foot land farther in front of you.

The old-school way of doing butt kicks was to keep your upper leg almost vertical and curl your heel around in a big arc until it hit your butt (figure 16.9*a*). However, this is not how you run, so it's not how you should practice running. Instead, the preferred way to do this drill is to bring your heel up toward the bottom of your butt in as straight a line as possible (figure 16.9*b*). When you do this, your knee will rise and your upper leg will move more parallel to the ground (though not to the extent seen in the high knees drill). This will start to sound familiar, but be sure to coordinate your arm with the opposite leg, land on your forefoot, and stand tall at all times. And as with the high knees drill, a progression from marching to skipping to running is an effective way to become familiar with the movement. Once again, perform short sets, prioritizing form at all times.

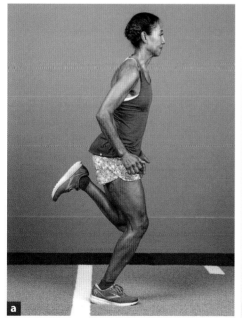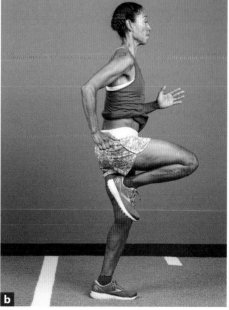

Figure 16.9　Butt kicks: *(a)* old school; *(b)* new school.

Straight-Leg Bounding

Straight-leg bounding is a great way to minimize your ground contact time and discourage overstriding, which can lead to injury. To execute straight-leg bounding, stand tall, keep a soft bend in your knees, and dorsiflex your ankle. Without increasing the bend in your knees—therefore, only hinging at your hips—use a scissors-kick motion to bound forward (figure 16.10). Focus on using your glutes to forcefully extend your hips and push off the ground. Note the sensation of your foot landing on its way back and under your center of gravity. Because you're eliminating movement at the knee joint, this will likely feel awkward at first, but if you stick with it, you'll gain confidence and then power. As with high knees, a common mistake is to lean back—don't do this! Your torso should be tall and upright as you do your straight-leg bounds.

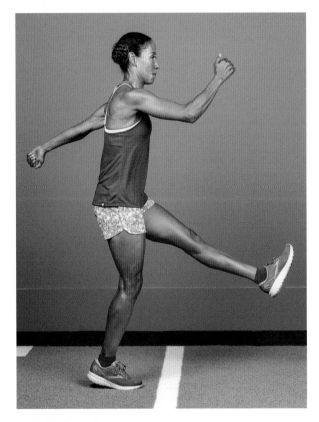

Figure 16.10   Straight-leg bounding.

Carioca (Grapevine)

Most running is performed straight ahead, or in the sagittal plane. Ironically, one way to ensure that your efforts are translating to forward motion rather than wasted lateral motion is to do some work in the frontal, or side-to-side, plane. This is effective because it helps stabilize your legs and avoid knee, lower back, and hip pain that can come from weak and unstable hips. It also helps you run more efficiently by wasting less motion. The carioca drill—also referred to as the grapevine drill—is one such drill that practices motion in the frontal plane. This drill targets the abductors and adductors.

To perform the carioca, move sideways, alternating crossing your trail leg (the one furthest from the direction you're moving) in front of you on one stride, and behind you on the next (figure 16.11). Be sure to keep your head and shoulders as squared up as possible; you should be twisting primarily from your hips. Do the drill in one direction for 10 to 15 seconds, rest, and then return in the other direction.

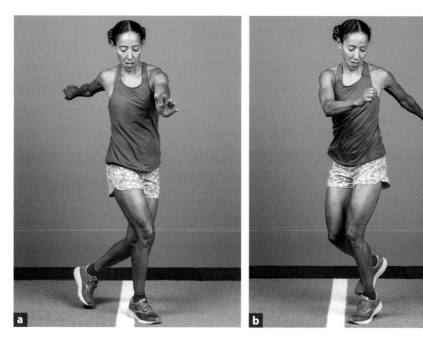

Figure 16.11   Carioca: *(a)* cross leg in front; *(b)* cross leg behind.

Strides

Strictly speaking, strides (or striders) are not really a drill, so much as they're just fast running. But they're effective at improving your form, nonetheless.

Strides are short sprints that allow you to "feel" good form for a short, controlled period. All runners look different—and in most cases better—when running fast than when running slow. The issue is that we don't have the physiology to support holding that fast pace for very long. Strides give us a little sample of the biomechanics of fast running and are therefore valuable for improving form. The goal is to teach your brain and body to run fast and with good form, so they are not treated as a conditioning exercise; they're meant to help your brain and your body learn how to communicate and cooperate when it's time to turn on the gas. They can be done on their own, as part of a drill set, or as part of longer runs. Throwing in a few strides late in a long run is an effective way to work on maintaining form even when fatigued.

Because of the neuromuscular focus, strides should be kept short. If your form deteriorates, stop the stride. Whether done on their own or as part of a longer run, the preferred method is to gradually work your speed up for five seconds or so and then keep that speed for another 10 to 15 seconds before slowing down.

Upper-Body Drill

If there were a contest for least-impressive-looking drill, this one would top the podium. But while you won't wow onlookers, practicing the upper-body drill can help the efficiency of your stride by increasing your kinesthetic sense, or your awareness of your body's position and movement, and decreasing wasted movement.

To do the upper-body drill, sit on the ground facing a mirror, with your legs extended straight in front of you. Sit nice and tall and begin mimicking the arm swing you'd do while running (figure 16.12). Watch yourself in the mirror and notice what you're doing. Are your hands crossing your midline? Are you shrugging your shoulders? As you speed up the drill, is your jaw tightening or are your arms unnecessarily tense? Are you pivoting from your shoulders while keeping your elbows at a fairly constant 90 degrees? (If you're not, you'll probably find out because your hand will come into contact with the ground.)

Do the movement for 20 to 30 seconds, observing yourself in the mirror. Does what you see in the mirror look like what you saw in your mind's eye? Now continue the movement, but close your eyes for 20 to 30 seconds before reopening them. Does it still look the same? If not, you'll start to get a sense of what your body is doing when you can't see it in a mirror and will increase your ability to self-correct when out in the real world.

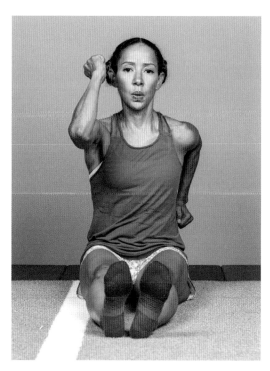

Figure 16.12   Upper-body drill.

Conclusion

To sum things up, there is no such thing as ideal form, and just because a runner is faster than you, that doesn't mean that you should emulate their form. However, there are many ways in which form modifications—which you can make by practicing drills two or three times per week—can make you a faster, more economical, and more resilient runner.

CHAPTER 17

Nutrition and Fueling

Virtually all athletes, coaches, and medical professionals will agree that good nutrition is essential to performance enhancement and overall health. On the other hand, the relationship between injuries and nutrition is often over-looked—yet it is vital. In this chapter we'll examine some eating practices, or as we like to call them fueling practices, that can help keep you healthy, on the road, and running strong.

RED-S and Eating Enough

To get some expert guidance on sports nutrition and how runners can eat to stay healthy, we spoke with Lauren Antonucci, MS, RDN, CSSD, CDE, CDN. For decades, Antonucci has helped keep endurance athletes performing at their best and is the author of *High-Performance Nutrition for Masters Athletes*. Fully expecting to hear her discuss the latest and greatest in supplements and ergogenic aids, exact formulas for hydrating during exercise, and other such topics, it was surprising but enlightening to hear her succinct, somewhat blunt guidance on what runners should eat: "Enough!"

According to the International Society of Sports Nutrition's position paper on Relative Energy Deficiency in Sport, or RED-S (Mountjoy et al. 2018), athletes should consume 30 kilocalories (what we think of as *calories*) per kilogram of lean mass. There's a good reason for this recommendation. Not only can underfueling lead to a whole host of health risks, it can lead to injury, too. For instance, research has found that an athlete who is not consuming sufficient calories relative to their caloric expenditure is four-and-a-half times more likely to suffer from a bone injury (Heikura et al. 2018).

You might be familiar with the term *female athlete triad*, which is a disordered eating pattern in which women underfuel relative to their energy needs, develop amenorrhea, and subsequently have a decrease in bone density, which can lead to stress fractures and other related issues. Though the first step of the triad—the disordered undereating—and subsequent bone density issues are more common in women than in men, they are not unique to women. By that same token, the consequences with respect to both overall health and running performance are also not exclusive to women. As a result, the more comprehensive and inclusive term RED-S has come into favor.

One of the particularly challenging aspects of RED-S is that, in the short term, the behaviors associated with the condition may in fact enhance performance. With all things being equal, a reduction in weight will often lead to faster race times. Unfortunately, those short-term gains mask the problem and often encourage the pattern of disordered eating to continue. Eventually, as the pattern of caloric deficit continues, the performance improvements do not. Chronic underfueling has potentially dangerous consequences that go well beyond slower race times. For instance, women will often stop menstruating, a condition called amenorrhea that results from hormonal dysregulation caused by insufficient caloric intake. It can result in fertility issues and osteoporosis. Meanwhile, anyone with the condition can suffer from long-term complications with their endocrine system; bone health; and cardiovascular, metabolic, and gastrointestinal functions (Korsten-Reck 2016).

Thus, before we take a deeper dive into micro- and macronutrients, the first factor to consider is whether an athlete is getting the necessary caloric intake to fuel their training and overall good health. As Antonucci firmly stated, "The rest is important only if you eat enough first." This may sound overly simplistic, but a good way to ensure that you're fueling adequately is that you should eat when you're hungry. Regularly failing to do so will leave you underfueled.

Macronutrients: Fats, Proteins, and Carbs

Nutrients are broken down into two categories, macronutrients and micronutrients. Macronutrients—fats, proteins, and carbohydrates—are the nutrients that provide the body with calories, or energy. Each serves its own nutritional purpose for humans.

Fats

In spite of what marketers and magazines of the last several decades might have you believe, fats are a necessary component of a healthy diet. Fat provides *essential* fatty acids, with that word *essential* referring to something that the body needs but cannot make at all or in sufficient quantity, and that therefore must be consumed. Fat helps the absorption of vitamin A, vitamin D, and vitamin E, all of which are necessary for growth, reproduction, and general health. Fats can help decrease inflammation and aid in hormone production. In short, fats are not the enemy.

Most of the time, opt for food choices that contain mono- and polyunsaturated fats (so-called good fats), but there is no reason to be fat-phobic with respect to your diet. In fact, according to the Academy of Nutrition and Dietetics Position Paper on Nutrition and Athletic Performance (Thomas, Erdman, and Burke 2016), 20 to 35 percent of daily calories should come from fat. Furthermore, they point out that decreasing fat intake to less than 20 percent has not been shown to benefit athletic performance.

Proteins

Protein is also high on the list of misunderstood macronutrients. Protein serves many purposes for athletes: It helps repair muscle tissue, it facilitates certain bodily functions such as digestion and water retention, and it keeps your immune system functioning at its peak, among many other roles. While there certainly can be some complications from excessive protein intake, there's an abundance of evidence that the recommended dietary allowance (RDA) for protein, a modest 0.8 grams per kilogram of body weight, is insufficient for athletes (Delimaris 2013). (In their efforts to build more muscle, strength athletes seem to have realized this long ago, but an endurance athlete's protein needs are similarly high.) Antonucci says that it's rare for an athlete to need less than 1.2 grams per kilogram, and she usually favors closer to 1.6. Moreover, in the case of injury, the needs may be even higher to reduce muscle loss and repair damaged tissue.

Voicing a common concern, one of Coach Cane's athletes once asked him whether too much protein could cause her to become too muscular, like some of the big guys she'd seen on magazine covers. Understandably, she didn't want to put on unnecessary muscle, which would weigh her down on runs. Coach Cane pointed out that doing a relatively short strength routine two or three times per week and fueling with adequate protein was not going to get her on the cover of *Muscle & Fitness* magazine any more than a couple of lessons with Serena Williams' coach would have her on center court at next year's U.S. Open. The truth is that protein alone will not build muscle. Without a sufficient stimulus (along with other factors), all the protein in the world won't make muscles grow. Weightlifters, powerlifters, bodybuilders, and other strength athletes provide that stimulus in the weight room through repeated intense lifting, and they generally also have a genetic makeup that encourages such growth. For a runner, accidentally becoming too muscular is not a likely outcome.

Carbs

Although carbohydrates have been vilified by some people in recent years, they should still be the primary source of calories in any endurance athlete's diet. Carbs provide the body's main source of energy. Most get broken down into glucose for use as fuel for your organs, particularly your brain, kidneys, and heart. When those organs are satiated, excess glucose can be stored in your muscles and liver in the form of glycogen, for quick and easy access later. While fats and even proteins *can* be used to fuel exercise, they are far less efficient than glycogen, which is why marathoners have historically "carb-loaded" prior to their races. (We now know enough to assure athletes that they don't need to pound numerous plates of pasta the night before their race, but it is worth being mindful of consuming simple carbohydrates leading up to the race, to make sure your glycogen stores are fully topped up.)

Low-carb diets have come into favor in recent years because some people think they are a great way to lose weight quickly. However, the ugly truth is that the fast results people see aren't due to shedding unwanted fat, they're due to shedding water. Glycogen holds approximately three times its weight in water (Fernandez-Elias et al. 2015); therefore, depleting glycogen stores, which can be upwards of 2,000 grams, can result in a big dip in the scale, but it will negatively impact your performance, since you are, in essence, dehydrating yourself. As Coach Cane likes to remind his athletes, "You're a distance runner, not a contestant on *The Biggest Loser.*"

Macronutrients for Recovery

One of the most effective ways to both improve performance and decrease the risk of injuries and illness is to recover by fueling properly—and adequately—after runs. Both carbohydrates and protein are crucial for optimal recovery. As mentioned earlier in the chapter, protein is necessary for muscle repair, regeneration, and synthesis, while carbohydrates are necessary to replenish the glycogen you used up during your run.

The recommended quantity of these macronutrients depends on the duration and intensity of your workout, as well as your age. Generally, athletes under 30 years old should shoot for 15 to 20 grams of protein shortly after a run, complemented by 0.5 grams of carbohydrate per kilogram (or 2.2 pounds) of body weight. So, a 27-year-old woman who weighs 59 kilograms (about 130 pounds) ought to consume 15 to 20 grams of protein and about 30 grams of carbohydrate. There is increasing evidence that protein requirements change as athletes age, so for masters runners, protein needs after prolonged or intense exercise may be as high as 30 to 40 grams to help muscle synthesis and avoid muscle degradation. Ideally, these calories should be ingested shortly after exercise to maximize their effect and to promote glycogen replenishment—within 15 to 20 minutes is ideal, and within two hours is necessary for best effect.

If you can't tolerate solid food after a run, there are plenty of options for homemade or commercially prepared recovery drinks and shakes. Chocolate milk gets lots of attention as a low-frills, low-cost option, but if that's not your preference, you have several choices for liquid recovery foods, and even a basic fruit-and-yogurt smoothie can get the job done.

Micronutrients: Vitamins and Minerals

Collectively, vitamins and minerals are referred to as micronutrients. Each micronutrient plays a unique role in overall health and well-being, but for the purposes of injury prevention and recovery, a few are of particular importance. Those are iron, calcium, vitamin D, and zinc.

Iron

Iron is a super-important element for runners. It's part of hemoglobin, which is the red blood cell molecule that transports oxygen to the working muscles (and elsewhere).

Inadequate iron intake can contribute to a variety of issues that can impair a runner's health and performance, including anemia, decrease in bone density, and immunosuppression. While in many cases vitamin and mineral supplementation is frivolous, iron supplementation is recommended by the American College of Sports Medicine and other credible organizations (Zourdos, Sanchez-Gonzalez, and Mahoney 2015).

When a runner complains of low energy levels, an iron deficiency *could* be to blame. Because the daily iron requirements for premenopausal women is 18 milligrams, as opposed to eight milligrams for men, low iron is of particular concern for premenopausal women, and nearly half of female athletes are iron deficient (Killip, Bennett, and Chambers 2007). (It's not unheard of for men to be deficient, but the prevalence is much lower.) If you are feeling perpetually fatigued despite getting adequate rest, have an unusually high resting heart rate, or notice that your skin, gums, and nails are paler than usual, it may be worth seeing a doctor to have your iron levels checked.

Calcium

Most people know that calcium is vital to bone health and is stored in the bones, but calcium serves a metabolic purpose, as well. When an athlete fails to consume enough calcium, the calcium that's stored in bones gets used for the metabolic role, thus weakening the bones and leaving the athlete at risk for stress fractures and other bone-related issues. This is why it's important to eat enough, overall, and to eat enough calcium, specifically.

As with many other nutrients, the amount of calcium a person requires varies depending on age. According to the National Academy of Science's Food and Nutrition Board, teenage and senior runners require more (1,300 and 1,200 milligrams per day, respectively) than adults (1,000 milligrams per day; Institute of Medicine [US] Standing Committee on the Scientific Evaluation of Dietary Reference Intakes 1997). Other conditions and factors can affect a runner's calcium needs. At the start of this chapter we discussed RED-S and the dangers of amenorrhea. Amenorrhea can lead to low calcium levels because calcium is leeched from the bones, so a runner who is amenorrheic likely requires even more calcium than her menstruating counterpart.

Since the human body can't produce its own calcium, it needs to be ingested from other sources such as dairy products, dark leafy vegetables, and fish with edible bones. Many foods, such as cereals and fruit juices, are fortified with calcium. Supplementation may be necessary if your diet is deficient in calcium, but there is growing evidence that calcium supplementation is not nearly as effective (if it is effective at all) as consuming it through natural food sources (Johns Hopkins Medicine n.d.).

Vitamin D

Vitamin D is obtained from food—particularly fatty fish, but also mushrooms, cheese, and egg yolk (National Institutes of Health 2020)—and from the sun. If you think about vitamin D in your diet at all, you probably think of its role in the regulation of calcium and bone mineralization. However, it also helps with cell growth and immune function. Because of its multiple roles, runners must get adequate vitamin D to stay healthy and injury-free. A variety of factors can lead to low vitamin D levels, including dark skin, living far from the equator, being indoors a lot, low dairy and fish intake, and being elderly or overweight. Supplementation may be appropriate if your diet and sun exposure are not adequate.

Zinc

While zinc is not necessarily directly helpful in injury prevention, it does play a role in keeping illness at bay, because it is essential for a healthy immune system. There is evidence that running (and other endurance exercise) decreases the body's zinc levels, which may be one reason runners are susceptible to illness and infection after hard efforts (Cordova and Alvarez-Mon 1995). Ensuring adequate zinc intake—ideally through eating foods like oysters, clams, liver, wheat germ, and fortified breakfast cereals, but alternately via supplementation—can help a runner's overall health. Men and women should strive to consume 11 and 8 milligrams per day, respectively (Institute of Medicine [US] Panel on Micronutrients 2001).

Conclusion

The information from this chapter should be enough to get you started in your efforts to use nutrition to help prevent or recover from injuries, but it is far from exhaustive. If you choose to seek further professional guidance, keep in mind that the credential Registered Dietitian (RD) is legally protected and requires board certification, while "nutritionist" is far less stringent and meaningful. In fact, some states allow the use of the title of nutritionist with no formal education. The Academy of Nutrition and Dietetics is a good resource for finding a qualified professional, and we—as well as the American College of Sports Medicine—recommend specifically looking for a board-certified specialist in sports dietetics (CSSD).

CHAPTER 18

Alternative Therapies and Myth Busting

Australian humorist Tim Minchin once said, "You know what they call alternative medicine that's been proved to work? Medicine." While that was said as a joke, there's a lot of truth to it. Many so-called alternative treatments lack empirical evidence to support them, instead relying on some combination of celebrity and athlete endorsements and pseudoscience. Some alternative therapies are appealing because they're perceived as new or cutting edge, while others benefit from the aura of thousands of years of use.

Regardless, the placebo effect—which is a beneficial effect that's due to a person's belief that a treatment will help them, rather than due to the treatment itself—is real and cannot be entirely dismissed. After all, the brain is a powerful organ, and while it cannot heal a broken bone for example, it absolutely impacts how we experience pain. Moreover, science is always evolving, and it would be unwise to summarily dismiss every new idea as nonsense.

With all of that in mind, let's take a look at some of the more prominent alternative treatments that have gained traction over the last several years and try to separate fact from fiction.

Cupping

In the 2016 Summer Olympics, countless athletes were seen with round discolorations all over their bodies. Given that one of those athletes was swimmer Michael Phelps, who would go on to win five gold medals that year, widespread interest arose around what these marks meant and how they might have aided Phelps' performance.

Those marks were the aftereffects of a technique known as cupping, which we mentioned in chapter 14 as a method of myofascial decompression. Cupping is the practice of placing glass cups against the skin to form a partial vacuum, which lifts the skin. It is thought this stimulates the circulation of blood to the area. This technique can be traced back thousands of years to China, Egypt, and the Middle East. Proponents claim it can help with issues such as pain and inflammation, can improve blood flow, and can assist in the removal of "toxins."

Does It Work?

Advocates are quick to point to Phelps and other world-class athletes who swear by the treatment. Still, the actual mechanism by which cupping therapy is supposed to work is unclear. While some studies have shown benefits ranging from improvements in blood cholesterol levels to pain relief (Yuan et al. 2015), most peer-reviewed science is not as supportive of the technique's efficacy. Designing double-blind studies (in which both the investigator and the subject are unaware of whether the technique in question or a placebo is being used) is hard when researching something like cupping, and most of the evidence used to argue in favor of cupping comes from studies that pair it with another treatment or have other biases. Much of the benefit seen may be attributed to the placebo effect (Charles et al. 2019).

Is It Safe?

Other than the telltale bruising, side effects are fairly minimal, though some instances of burning have also been observed (Jing-Chun et al. 2014).

Should I?

For the most part, the scientific community does not support cupping. Evidence-based practitioners point out that its advocates rely on anecdotal evidence and the placebo effect. While cupping alone is not going to propel you to the next Olympic games, cupping as a tool in soft tissue mobilization has been found to be clinically beneficial. Dr. Aguillard has used a combination of hard, plastic cups and soft, silicon cups in her physical therapy practice to help increase fascial glide in areas of the body that are very restricted. Cupping, or in physical therapy terminology, "myofascial decompression," is an effective alternative to traditional compression therapies, much in the way that Graston, or instrument-assisted tools, have been used. This technique is especially useful in areas of the body that have very dense connective tissue such as the IT band and the thoracolumbar fascia. Dr. Aguillard does not just put the cup on and walk away; the cup is lifted and pulled gently away from the skin and then glided across the surface to help separate the tissue or is accompanied with active movements, like a squat or a cat/cow, to facilitate tissue mobility.

Whole Body Cryotherapy

Whole body cryotherapy (WBC) is a technique in which your body is enclosed in a chamber and exposed to extremely cold air for two to four minutes. The term *cryotherapy* simply means cold therapy, and WBC is, as the name suggests, a means of delivering that therapy to the whole body rather than a localized area, as with an ice pack.

Does It Work?

Advocates claim WBC can help with everything from migraines to weight loss, arthritis pain to mood disorders, low-risk tumors to Alzheimer's. However, the suggestion that its efficacy is any greater or wider ranging than simpler, more traditional administration of cold therapy is dubious at best.

According to Aron Yustein, MD, a medical officer in the Food and Drug Administration's (FDA) Center for Devices and Radiological Health, "Based on purported health benefits seen in many promotions for cryotherapy spas, consumers may incorrectly believe that the FDA has cleared or approved WBC devices as safe and effective to treat medical conditions. . . . That is not the case" (U.S. FDA 2016). A review of research on WBC by Costello et al. (2015) failed to find sufficient evidence that WBC reduces self-reported muscle soreness or improves subjective recovery after exercise. In other words, the research just is not there to support this intervention.

Is It Safe?

Rashes, burns, and frostbite are among the potential side effects of WBC. Fatalities have occurred when this therapy is used improperly and unsupervised. For instance, in 2015, a cryotherapy spa worker was using the chamber unsupervised and either accidentally locked herself in or passed out. She was found dead 10 hours later (Helsel 2015).

Should I?

As with many other showy techniques, there's a certain "cool factor" to WBC (pun intended). But there's reason to be wary of claims that this technique is any more beneficial than an ice pack, ice bath, or other cold therapy that physical therapists, physicians, and athletic trainers have been using for decades.

Acupuncture

Acupuncture is a centuries-old method of treating pain, along with many other ailments, and is considered a staple of traditional Chinese medicine. It involves the insertion of very thin needles through the patient's skin at specific points on the body. The theory behind acupuncture is that it balances the patient's chi, or energy, which flows through specific pathways in the body. The insertion of needles into precise areas along this path is said to allow the practitioner to balance that flow.

Does It Work?

As is often the case, it depends whom you ask. On the one hand, it is widely used not only in Asia but across the United States and elsewhere, including within more conventional medical settings. On the other hand, the vast majority of peer-reviewed studies offer reason for skepticism. Simulated acupuncture, which involves randomly placing needles, rather than inserting them at precise sites, has shown comparable results to traditional acupuncture (Cherkin et al. 2009). Similarly, studies in which the subject is unable to view the insertion have shown that poking, but not breaking, the skin with toothpicks produces similar results (Cherkin et al. 2009). The Mayo Clinic points out "there's also evidence that acupuncture works best in people who expect it to work"—which is a strong argument for the placebo effect (Toroborg 2018).

Is It Safe?

When working with a certified practitioner who uses sterile needles, acupuncture is safe. There is very little risk of infection, and pain is usually minimal.

Should I?

Many people classify acupuncture in the "what's the harm?" category. When done by a trained acupuncturist, the answer is almost definitely "no harm." Whether it will be of any benefit remains an outstanding question.

Acupuncture Versus Dry Needling

While traditional acupuncture is up for debate, the clinical use of needles in trigger point therapy is very popular in the sports-rehab setting. You might find an acupuncturist who specializes in trigger point acupuncture or a physical therapist trained in dry needling—it's incredibly similar. Medical doctors also use trigger-point injections of lidocaine or saline to treat various conditions.

The overall technique involves inserting a thin needle directly into a trigger point, a point of tension within the musculoskeletal system (think of that really annoying knot in your upper trap or calf that just doesn't seem to go away). Like many other manual techniques, the goal is to send a signal to your nervous system to relax tension in a specific area by eliciting a twitch response (Vulfsons, Ratmansky, and Kalichman 2012).

Is dry needling the greatest manual therapy? No. If you're up for it, some heavy-duty work with your lacrosse ball can probably produce a similar effect. However, if you have some pesky points of tension that aren't responding to other treatments, dry needling could be worth a try.

Cannabidiol (CBD)

CBD, which is often used for pain relief as well as anxiety and sleep issues, is one of the most misunderstood treatments in this chapter. CBD is one of hundreds of chemical compounds contained in cannabis (i.e., marijuana). And while marijuana does cause users to get high, it is tetrahydrocannabinol (THC), not CBD, that produces the sensation. Moreover, a vast majority of CBD "health products" derive their CBD not from marijuana but from hemp, which is a related but entirely different plant.

Does It Work?

The evidence that CBD can help with childhood epilepsy seems promising (Ben-Zeev 2020). Similarly, the compound's effects on sleep and anxiety are also encouraging (Shannon et al. 2019). The claims that it can treat chronic pain are less convincing and still unproven.

There are sometimes concerns about an athlete testing positive for drugs from CBD. In theory, that should not happen because CBD is typically made from hemp rather than marijuana and therefore should be free of THC, the component of marijuana that creates a high. As long as the CBD product used is derived from hemp and there is no cross contamination or mislabeling, athletes shouldn't need to worry about a positive drug test from its use.

Is It Safe?

Nausea, fatigue, and irritability are listed as the most common side effects from CBD use and are relatively infrequent. The Mayo Clinic has also expressed concerns for those taking blood thinners, because CBD can interact with some other medications (Bauer 2020). Because CBD is classified as a supplement rather than a medication, FDA regulations are far looser, leading to some concerns about the consistency and quality control of CBD products.

Should I?

While many of the other treatments in this chapter have been studied for decades, CBD has not. It's certainly not the end-all-be-all that some would have you believe, but if you're dealing with chronic pain or struggle with sleep or anxiety—which can most certainly have a detrimental effect on your training—this is a treatment that may be worth investigating further.

Magnetic Therapy

For years, magnetic therapy of various types has been touted to improve a variety of health conditions, including pain. Generally, these claims have come from those trying to sell magnetic bracelets, insoles, or other paraphernalia, rather than from scientific and reputable sources.

Does It Work?

Though its persistent marketing would suggest otherwise, the overwhelming preponderance of scientific evidence says no (Basford 2001).

Is It Safe?

Those who have a pacemaker or an insulin pump or are pregnant should steer clear to stay on the safe side (Heart Rhythm Society 2006). Everyone else is probably in the clear.

Should I?

In a word, no. In a few more words, magnetic therapy advocates have hypothesized a variety of mechanisms by which this therapy could be beneficial but have consistently failed to prove any of them. So save your money for something else.

Detoxes and Cleanses

Detoxification (detox) diets or cleanses are touted as a way rid your body of "toxins," resulting in a "cleaner," more efficient athlete. The exact detox protocols vary; most advocate a period of fasting followed by a restricted diet of some combination of juices, raw vegetables, and often nutritional supplements.

Does It Work?

For humans who possess a functioning liver, lungs, skin, and at least one kidney, detoxes and cleanses add no value. Those organs require no boost or assistance to rid your body of unwanted material and are best left alone to do their job. In fact, according to pharmacist Scott Gavura, "There is no credible evidence to demonstrate that detox kits do anything at all. They have not been shown to remove 'toxins' or offer any health benefits" (Gavura 2015).

Is It Safe?

Some detoxes include more invasive methods such as coffee enemas, which come with their own safety concerns (Son et al. 2020). Otherwise, they're likely safe if used for short periods of time.

Should I?

Hardly. Refer to the nutrition chapter, where rule number one was "eat enough." Depriving yourself of necessary nutrients in a futile and unnecessary attempt to cleanse your body is useless, at best, and counterproductive at worst.

Infrared Saunas

Traditional saunas have been around for thousands of years. Typically they use charcoal or stones to heat a room, causing anyone shut inside to heat up and eventually sweat. Infrared saunas (or far-infrared saunas) rely on infrared light, which is purported to heat the body from the inside out, therefore requiring far lower temperatures than in traditional saunas (around 135 degrees Fahrenheit versus 185 degrees Fahrenheit or more). Some advocates of infrared saunas suggest that their mechanism is more effective for removal of heavy metals or other "toxins." Others suggest that the simple fact that it's more comfortable than traditional saunas allows the user to tolerate it for a longer period of time, thereby increasing its efficacy.

Does It Work?

As with many other health trends, those promoting infrared saunas make vague health claims, reference unnamed "toxins," and rely heavily on celebrity testimonials. Meanwhile, as in so many cases, scientific consensus is equivocal at best. Some studies have shown benefits for chronic health conditions, and some have suggested modest cardiovascular benefits in untrained populations (Laukkanen, Khan, and Zaccardi 2015). Some people may also like it to help with heat acclimatization if they're training for a hot weather race while living in a cooler climate. However, the notion that a sauna of any type will help you sweat out toxins to any significant degree is not backed by science.

Is It Safe?

If you're pregnant, lactating, or have cardiovascular disease, you may want to err on the side of being overly cautious and avoid saunas. Otherwise, saunas—infrared or otherwise—appear to be safe.

Should I?

When Coach Cane was a child and contracted a cold, his grandmother insisted he eat her delicious, homemade chicken soup. When he asked her if it would help his cold, her response was "it can't hurt." Think of saunas as the chicken soup of wellness: You may enjoy them, and they may make you feel a little better, but be wary if someone claims they have magic properties.

Conclusion

When Mark Spitz was setting the swimming world on fire, he told a Soviet coach that his improvement was due in part to his newly grown and soon-to-be trademark mustache. He claimed that the Americans had done extensive testing, and that the facial hair made him more hydrodynamic, promoting faster times in the pool. Months later when he encountered the Soviets at another meet, they had all grown moustaches. Of course, Spitz's gold-medal performances were due to countless hours of conditioning and endless laps spent refining his stroke technique; they had nothing to do with his mustache.

Similarly, if a runner is faster than you, it's highly likely that it's due to some combination of genetics, training, and experience—not the pills or drinks or jelly beans they're endorsing. So when a new treatment comes across your radar, remember that scientific proof doesn't come from anecdotes, no matter how numerous or high-profile. Instead, as with nearly everything we've recommended in this book, check with your doctor or other trusted (licensed) health professional for guidance.

References

Antonucci, L.A. 2021. *High-Performance Nutrition for Masters Athletes*. Chicago, IL: Human Kinetics.

Asplund, C.A., and T.M. Best. 2013. Achilles tendon disorders. *The BMJ* 346: f1262.

Basford, J.R. 2001. A historical perspective of the popular use of electric and magnetic therapy. *Archives of Physical Medicine and Rehabilitation* 82(9).

Bass, E. 2012. Tendinopathy: Why the difference between tendinitis and tendinosis matters. *International Journal of Therapeutic Massage & Bodywork* 5(1): 14-17.

Bauer, B.A. 2020. "What are the benefits of CBD—and is it safe to use?" Mayo Clinic. December 18, 2020. https://www.mayoclinic.org/healthy-lifestyle/consumer-health/expert-answers/is-cbd-safe-and-effective/faq-20446700.

Beatty, N.R., I. Félix, J. Hettler, P.J. Moley, and J.F. Wyss. 2017. Rehabilitation and prevention of proximal hamstring tendinopathy. *Current Sports Medicine Reports* 16(3): 162-171.

Beer, B. 2019. Hamstring strength for runners. *POGO Physio*. https://www.pogophysio.com.au/blog/hamstring-strength-for-runners/.

Ben-Zeev, B. 2020. Medical cannabis for intractable epilepsy in childhood: A review. *Rambam Maimonides Medical Journal* 11(1): e0004.

Bourne, M.N., S. Duhig, R. Timmins, M. Williams, D.A. Opar, A. Al Najjar, G.K. Kerr, and A. Shield. 2017. Impact of the Nordic hamstring and hip extension exercises on hamstring architecture and morphology: Implications for injury prevention. *British Journal of Sports Medicine* 51 (5): 469-477.

Camasta, C.A. 1996. Hallux limitus and hallux rigidus. Clinical examination, radiographic findings, and natural history. *Clinics in Podiatric Medicine and Surgery* 13 (3): 423-448.

Charles D.,T. Hudgins, J. MacNaughton, E. Newman, J. Tan, and M. Wigger. 2019. A systematic review of manual therapy techniques, dry cupping and dry needling in the reduction of myofascial pain and myofascial trigger points. *Journal of Bodywork and Movement Therapies* 3 (3): 539-546.

Chaudhry, H., R. Schleip, Z. Ji, B. Bukiet, M. Maney, and T. Findley. 2008. Three-dimensional mathematical model for deformation of human fasclae in manual therapy. *The Journal of the American Osteopathic Association* 108: 379-390.

Cheatham, S.W., M.J. Kolber, M. Cain, and M. Lee. 2015. The effects of self-myofascial release using a foam roll or roller massager on joint range of motion, muscle recovery, and performance: A systematic review. *International Journal of Sports Physical Therapy* 10 (6): 827-838.

Cherkin, D.C., K.J. Sherman, A.L. Avins, J.H. Erro, L. Ichikawa, W.E. Barlow, K. Delaney, R. Hawkes, L. Hamilton, A. Pressman, P.S. Khalsa, and R.A. Deyo. 2009. A randomized trial comparing acupuncture, simulated acupuncture, and usual care for chronic low back pain. Archives of Internal Medicine 169(9): 858-866.

Colapietro, M., J.J. Fraser, J.E. Resch, and J. Hertel. 2020. Running mechanics during 1600 meter track runs in young adults with and without chronic ankle instability. *Physical Therapy in Sport* 42: 16-25.

Cordova, A., and M. Alvarez-Mon. 1995. Behaviour of zinc in physical exercise: A special reference to immunity and fatigue. *Neuroscience & Biobehavioral Reviews* 19 (3): 439-445.

Costello, J.T., P.R. Baker, G.M. Minett, F. Bieuzen, I.B. Stewart, and C. Bleakley. 2015. Whole-body cryotherapy (extreme cold air exposure) for preventing and treating muscle soreness after exercise in adults. *Cochrane Database of Systematic Reviews* 9.

Craib, M.W., V.A. Mitchell, K.B. Fields, T.R. Cooper, R. Hopewell, and D.W. Morgan. 1996. The association between flexibility and running economy in sub-elite male distance runners. *Medicine & Science in Sport & Exercise* 28 (6): 737-743.

Delimaris, I. 2013. Adverse effects associated with protein intake above the recommended dietary allowance for adults. *International Scholarly Research Notices*, 126929.

Fernandez-Elias, V.E., J.F. Ortega, R.K. Nelson, and R. Mora-Rodriguez. 2015. Relationship between muscle water and glycogen recovery after prolonged exercise in the heat in humans. *European Journal of Applied Physiology* 115 (9): 1919-1926.

Franklin, S., M.J. Grey, N. Heneghan, L. Bowen, and F-X Li. 2015. Barefoot vs common footwear: A systematic review of the kinematic, kinetic and muscle activity differences during walking. *Gait & Posture* 43 (3): 230-239.

Fredericson, M., and C. Wolf. 2005. Iliotibial band syndrome in runners: Innovations in treatment. *Sports Medicine* 35: 451-459.

Gavura, S. 2015." Detox: What 'they' don't want you to know." Science-Based Medicine. https://sciencebasedmedicine.org/detox-what-they-dont-want-you-to-know/

Haddad, M., A. Dridi, M. Chtara, A. Chaouachi, D. Wong, D. Behm, and K. Chamari. 2014. Static stretching can impair explosive performance for at least 24 hours. *Journal of Strength and Conditioning Research* 28 (1): 140-146.

Hadeed, A., and D.C. Tapscott. 2020. Iliotibial band friction syndrome. In *StatPearls*. Treasure Island, FL: StatPearls Publishing. https://www.ncbi.nlm.nih.gov/books/NBK542185/.

Han, J., J. Anson, G. Waddington, R. Adams, and Y. Liu. 2015. The role of ankle proprioception for balance control in relation to sports performance and injury. *BioMed Research International* 2015, 842804.

Hanc, J. 2015. Pat Petersen, a former U.S. Marathon record holder, dies at 55. *Runner's World*. June 1, 2015. https://www.runnersworld.com/news/a20805236/pat-petersen-a-former-u-s-marathon-record-holder-dies-at-55/.

Heart Rhythm Society. 2006. "Magnets may pose serious risks for patients with pacemakers and ICDs." ScienceDaily. November 30, 2006.

Heikura, I.A., A.L.T. Uusitalo, T. Stellingwerff, D. Bergland, A.A. Mero, and L.M. Burke. 2018. Low energy availability is difficult to assess but outcomes have large impact on bone injury rates in elite distance athletes. *International Journal of Sport Nutrition and Exercise Metabolism* 28 (4): 403-411.

Helsel, P. 2015. Nevada spa worker suffocated in cryochamber, coroner rules. NBC News, November 10, 2015. https://www.nbcnews.com/news/us-news/nevada-spa-worker-suffocated-cryochamber-coroner-rules-n461111.

Herbert, R.D., M. de Noronha, and S.J. Kamper. 2011. Stretching to prevent or reduce muscle soreness after exercise. *Cochrane Database of Systematic Reviews* 6 (7).

Hoffman, M.D., N. Badowski, J. Chin, and K.J. Stuempfle. 2016. A randomized controlled trial of massage and pneumatic compression for ultramarathon recovery. *Journal of Orthopaedic & Sports Physical Therapy* 46 (5): 320-326.

Institute of Medicine (US) Panel on Micronutrients. 2001. *Dietary Reference Intakes for Vitamin A, Vitamin K, Arsenic, Boron, Chromium, Copper, Iodine, Iron, Manganese, Molybdenum, Nickel, Silicon, Vanadium, and Zinc*. Washington, DC: National Academies Press.

Institute of Medicine (US) Standing Committee on the Scientific Evaluation of Dietary Reference Intakes. 1997. *Dietary Reference Intakes for Calcium, Phosphorus, Magnesium, Vitamin D, and Fluoride*. Washington, DC: National Academies Press.

Jafary, H. 2020. "What's the difference between bunions and big toe arthritis?" The Bunion Institute. https://www.bunioninstitute.com/blog/difference-between-bunion-and-big-toe-arthritis/.

Jing-Chun, Z., Y. Jia-Ao, X. Chun-Jing, S. Kai, and L. Lai-Jin. 2014. Burns induced by cupping therapy in a burn center in northeast China. *Wounds* 26 (7): 214-220.

Johns Hopkins Medicine. n.d. "Calcium supplements: Should you take them?" https://www.hopkinsmedicine.org/health/wellness-and-prevention/calcium-supplements-should-you-take-them.

Jones, B.H., and J.J. Knapik. 1999. Physical training and exercise-related injuries. Surveillance, research and injury prevention in military populations. *Sports Medicine* 27 (2): 111-125.

Jung, A.P. The impact of resistance training on distance running performance. 2003. *Sports Medicine* 33 (7): 539-552.

Killip, S., J.M. Bennett, and M.D. Chambers. 2007. Iron deficiency anemia: Evaluation and management. *American Family Physician* 75 (5): 671-678.

Korsten-Reck, U. 2016. The IOC Consensus Statement: Beyond the female athlete triad—Relative Energy Deficiency in Sports (RED-S). *Deutsche Zeitschrift Für Sportmedizin* 3: 68-71.

Laukkanen, T., H. Khan, F. Zaccardi. 2015. Association between sauna bathing and fatal cardiovascular and all-cause mortality events. *JAMA Internal Medicine* 175 (4): 542-548.

Lenhart, R., D. Thelen, and B. Heiderscheit. 2014. Hip muscle loads during running at various step rates. *Journal of Orthopaedic & Sports Physical Therapy* 44 (10): 766-A4.

Maselli, F., L. Storari, V. Barbari, A. Colombi, A. Turolla, S. Gianola, G. Rossettini, and M. Testa. 2020. Prevalence and incidence of low back pain among runners: A systematic review. *BMC Musculoskeletal Disorders* 21 (1): 343.

McDonald, K.A., S.M. Stearne, J.A. Alderson, I. North, N.J. Pires, and J. Rubenson. 2016. The role of arch compression and metatarsophalangeal joint dynamics in modulating plantar fascia strain in running. *PLoS One* 11 (4): e0152602.

Menzies, P., C. Menzies, L. McIntyre, P. Paterson, J. Wilson, and O.J. Kemi. 2010. Blood lactate clearance during active recovery after an intense running bout depends on the intensity of the active recovery. *Journal of Sports Science* 28 (9): 975-982.

Mirkin, G. 2020. "Why ice delays recovery." DrMirkin.com. Last modified June 6, 2020. https://www.drmirkin.com/fitness/why-ice-delays-recovery.html.

Moen, M.H., J.L. Tol, A. Weir, M. Steunebrink, and T.C. De Winter. 2009. Medial tibial stress syndrome: A critical review. *Sports Medicine* 39: 523-546.

Moore, K.L., A.F. Daly, and A.M.R. Agur. 2010. *Clinically Oriented Anatomy.* 6th ed. Baltimore: Lippincott Williams and Wilkins.

Moran, M.W., and K.R. Rogowski. 2020. Hip and pelvic stability and gait retraining in the management of athletic pubalgia and hip labral pathology in a female runner: A case report. *International Journal of Sports Physical Therapy* 15 (6): 1174-1183.

Mountjoy, M., J. Sundgot-Borgen, L. Burke, K.E. Ackerman, C. Blauwet, N. Constantini, C. Lebrun, et al. 2018. International Olympic Committee (IOC) Consensus Statement on Relative Energy Deficiency in Sport (RED-S): 2018 update. *International Journal of Sport Nutrition and Exercise Metabolism* 28 (4): 316-331.

National Institutes of Health. 2020. Vitamin D: Fact sheet for health professionals. Last modified October 9, 2020. https://ods.od.nih.gov/factsheets/VitaminD-HealthProfessional/.

Neumann, D.A. 2010. *Kinesiology of the Musculoskeletal System: Foundations for Rehabilitation.* 2nd ed. St. Louis, MO: Mosby/Elsevier.

Noehren, B., M.B. Pohl, Z. Sanchez, T. Cunningham, and C. Lattermann. 2012. Proximal and distal kinematics in female runners with patellofemoral pain. *Clinical Biomechanics,* 27 (4): 366-371.

Raabe, M.E., and A.M.W. Chaudhari. 2018. Biomechanical consequences of running with deep core muscle weakness. *Journal of Biomechanics* 67: 98-105.

Reuell, P. 2015. Understanding the IT band. *The Harvard Gazette,* August 26, 2015. https://news.harvard.edu/gazette/story/2015/08/understanding-the-it-band/.

Rio, E., K. Dawson, G. Lorimer Moseley, J. Gaida, S. Docking, C. Purdam, and J. Cook. 2016. Tendon neuroplastic training: Changing the way we think about tendon rehabilitation: A narrative review. *British Journal of Sports Medicine* 50: 209-215.

Rio E., D. Kidgell, C. Purdam, J. Gaida, G. Lorimer Moseley, A.J. Pearce, and J. Cook. 2015. Isometric exercise induces analgesia and reduces inhibition in patellar tendinopathy. *British Journal of Sports Medicine* 49: 1277-1283.

Schoenfeld, B., B. Contreras, J. Krieger, J. Grgic, K. Delcastillo, R. Belliard, and A. Alto. 2019. Resistance training volume enhances muscle hypertrophy but not strength in trained men. *Medicine & Science in Sport & Exercise* 51 (1): 94-103.

Schwane, J.A., B.G. Watrous, S.R. Johnson, and R.B. Armstrong. 1983. Is lactic acid related to delayed-onset muscle soreness? *The Physician and Sportsmedicine* 11 (3): 124-131.

Shannon, S., N. Lewis, H. Lee, and S. Hughes. 2019. Cannabidiol in anxiety and sleep: A large case series. *The Permanente Journal* 23: 18-41.

Son, H., H.J. Song, H.J. Seo, H. Lee, S.M. Choi, and S. Lee. 2020. The safety and effectiveness of self-administered coffee enema: A systematic review of case reports. *Medicine (Baltimore)* 99 (36): e21998.

Teng, H.L., and C.M. Powers. 2016. Hip-extensor strength, trunk posture, and use of the knee-extensor muscles during running. *Journal of Athletic Training* 51 (7): 519-524.

Thacker, S.B., J. Gilchrist, D.F. Stroup, and C. Dexter Kimsey. 2002. The prevention of shin splints in sports: A systematic review of literature. *Medicine & Science in Sports & Exercise* 34: 32-40.

Thacker. S.B., J. Gilchrist, D.F. Stroup, and C.D. Kimsey Jr. 2004. The impact of stretching on sports injury risk: A systematic review of the literature. *Medicine & Science in Sport & Exercise* 36 (3): 371-378.

Thomas, D.T., K.A. Erdman, and L.M. Burke. 2016. Position of the Academy of Nutrition and Dietetics, Dietitians of Canada, and the American College of Sports Medicine: Nutrition and athletic performance. *Journal of the Academy of Nutrition and Dietetics* 116 (3): 501-528.

Toroborg, L. 2018. "Mayo Clinic Q and A: Curious about acupuncture?" Mayo Clinic. Last modified April 20, 2018. https://newsnetwork.mayoclinic.org/discussion/mayo-clinic-q-and-a-curious-about-acupuncture/.

U.S. Food & Drug Administration. 2016. "Whole body cryotherapy (WBC): A 'cool' trend that lacks evidence, poses risks." Last modified July 5, 2016. https://www.fda.gov/consumers/consumer-updates/whole-body-cryotherapy-wbc-cool-trend-lacks-evidence-poses-risks.

van Gent, R.N., D. Siem, M. van Middelkoop, A.G. van Os, S.M.A Bierma-Zeinstra, and B.W. Koes. 2007. Incidence and determinants of lower extremity running injuries in long distance runners: A systematic review. *British Journal of Sports Medicine* 41: 469-480.

Vulfsons, S., M. Ratmansky, and L. Kalichman. 2012. Trigger point needling: Techniques and Outcome. *Current Pain and Headache Reports* 16 (5): 407-412.

Willy, R.W., M.T. Manal, E.E. Witvrouw, and I.S. Davis. 2012. Are mechanics different between male and female runners with patellofemoral pain? *Medicine & Science in Sports & Exercise* 44 (11): 2165-2171. https://doi.org/10.1249/MSS.0b013e3182629215.

Willy R.W., J.P. Scholz, and I.S. Davis. 2012. Mirror gait retraining for the treatment of patellofemoral pain in female runners. *Clinical Biomechanics* 27 (10): 1045-1051.

Wilson, J.M., L.M. Hornbuckle, J.S. Kim, C. Ugrinowitsch, S.R. Lee, M.C. Zourdos, B. Sommer, and L.B. Panton. 2010. Effects of static stretching on energy cost and running endurance performance. *Journal of Strength and Conditioning Research* 24 (9): 2274-2279.

Yuan, Q.L., T.M. Guo, L. Liu, F. Sun, and Y.G. Zhang. 2015. Traditional Chinese medicine for neck pain and low back pain: A systematic review and meta-analysis. *PLoS One* 24; 10 (2): e0117146.

Zourdos, M.C., M.A. Sanchez-Gonzalez, and S.E. Mahoney. 2015. A brief review: The implications of iron supplementation for marathon runners on health and performance. *Journal of Strength and Conditioning Research* 29 (2): 559-565.

Index

About the Authors

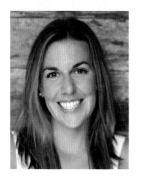

Emmi Aguillard, PT, DPT, FAFS, is a full-time physical therapist managing her own private practice that specializes in treating and training runners. She also has advanced training in pelvic health and works with women to maintain their optimal fitness during pregnancy and safely return to running after giving birth. Prior to that, she worked at Finish Line Physical Therapy in New York City.

Dr. Aguillard earned her doctorate of physical therapy from Columbia University after graduating from Tulane University, where she competed for the women's NCAA Division I track and field and cross country programs. She completed her fellowship in applied functional science through the Gray Institute and has taken numerous courses through the Postural Restoration Institute. Outside of her physical therapy practice, she coaches the 900-member Dashing Whippets running team, creating strength programs and team training plans for road races ranging from 5K to marathon, and she works with Matt Wilpers as a Team Wilpers coach. She has also been a contributing writer to *Women's Health and Cooking Light*.

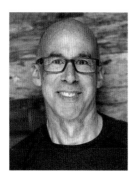

Jonathan Cane, better known as Coach Cane, has been coaching endurance athletes for over 30 years. He holds a master's degree in exercise physiology from Adelphi University and has coached for Nike, JackRabbit, and Under Armour. Cane is the coauthor of *Triathlon Anatomy* (Human Kinetics) as well as *The Complete Idiot's Guide to Weight Training*, and he has written for *Triathlete magazine*, *MetroSports Magazine*, *New York Runner*, and more. He has been a featured speaker for Nike, New York Road Runners, Chelsea Piers Triathlon Club, Hospital for Special Surgery, and others. He lives in the Bronx, New York, with his wife, triathlete Nicole Sin Quee; their son, Simon; and their pit bull, Lola.

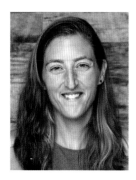

Allison Goldstein is a writer and editor who works with business leaders, award-winning academics, and professionals to bring their literary ideas to the world. She is also a competitive runner and raced in the 2020 Olympic Trials marathon. Her work has appeared in *Runner's World*, *Women's Running*, *Bicycling*, *Popular Mechanics*, and other publications. Goldstein is based in Jersey City, New Jersey.

You read the book—now complete the companion CE exam to earn continuing education credit!

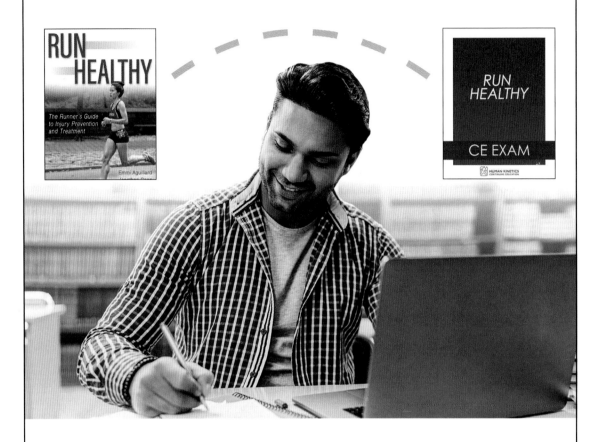

Find and purchase the companion CE exam here:
US.HumanKinetics.com/collections/CE-Exam
Canada.HumanKinetics.com/collections/CE-Exam

50% off the companion CE exam with this code

RH2024

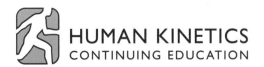